This book is dedicated to my mom.

Thank you for all the sacrifices you made to get me to where I am today.

Autism Wellbeing Plan:
How to Get Your Child Healthy

CHRISTIAN YORDANOV

The information in this book is intended for educational purposes only. It is based on the research and professional experience of the author and should not be taken as professional medical advice, nor is it to be used as a substitute for medical care. For medical advice, always consult your physician and get their approval before implementing dietary changes or beginning any nutritional supplements. All efforts have been made to assure the accuracy of the information contained in this book as of the date of publication. The author and publisher specifically disclaim all responsibility for any liability, loss or risk, personal or otherwise, that is incurred as a consequence, directly or indirectly, of the use and application of the contents of this book. The publisher is not responsible for websites (or their content) that are not owned by the publisher.

Published by Health Educo Ltd

Editor: James Barnett
Cover Design: Davor Dramikanin
Illustrations: Ivelina Ivanova

ISBN: 978-1-9163930-0-4
eISBN: 978-1-9163930-1-1

First Edition

CONTENTS

INTRODUCTION

Chances are high that if your child is diagnosed with an autism spectrum disorder (ASD), or you suspect they may be on the autistic spectrum, they are also experiencing one or more of the following health issues:

- Gastrointestinal problems (e.g. constipation, diarrhoea, abdominal pain, reflux, maldigestion, leaky gut)
- Gut infections (e.g. parasites, bacterial, or fungal)
- Food allergies or sensitivities
- Sleep problems
- Nutrient deficiencies or imbalances
- Impaired immune function
- Heavy metal or chemical toxicity

Most parents are not aware that nearly all of the above have been shown by researchers to correlate with autism severity. In other words, studies have shown health problems such as gut issues, bacterial infections, nutrient imbalances, heavy metal and chemical toxicity, and immune dysfunction to be associated with an increase in autistic symptoms.[1-22]

More importantly, these health issues are causing children, and their families, unneeded suffering. If your youngster can't sleep, you can't sleep. If they have tummy trouble, they are more likely to act out. An unhealthy child means more doctor visits and more cancelled plans. It means less fun times and more worries and frustrations.

Much of this suffering and frustration is avoidable because many of the issues above are not particularly difficult to correct or improve - if you know to look for them. This is exactly what I'd like to help you do.

With this book, I will teach you how to identify and address your child's health challenges, so that both of you can have a better quality of life.

I've scoured hundreds of scientific papers to find the information that is clearly not making its way to the majority of parents and doctors, and condensed it into easily understandable action items.

In the coming chapters, you will discover ways in which you can become more proactive about your child's health.

Will the autism symptoms improve? Every case is so unique that it's impossible to say. Oftentimes, as a person gets healthier, many of their symptoms do start to melt away. But that's not our goal here. As I will explain later, chasing symptoms and trying to suppress them is entirely the wrong strategy. What will improve is your child's health and wellbeing, and that, in my opinion, is the goal worthy of pursuit.

This Book is NOT About "Fixing Your Child"

Please don't interpret anything in this book as trying to "fix your child". There is nothing to fix! Your child is a wonderful human being with a unique character and qualities that this book is not looking to change. Rather, it is about allowing them to be their happiest and healthiest self.

But if your child had the flu or a stomach bug, would you not do something to help them? What if it was a sprained ankle or other injury? Of course you would! Surely as soon as you found out it had happened.

Now take a moment to think about this: let's say you ran a test that showed you that your child has harmful bacteria in their gut. Or you found out they have several nutrient deficiencies. Or they are eating foods that are harming them, or they are having trouble eliminating toxic metals or chemicals from their body.

Would you do something about it? I think most parents would answer with a resounding yes. Would you think that you were "trying to fix your child"? Surely not. You would simply be doing your job as a parent to resolve the issue and improve the quality of their life. Would you just sit back and accept the circumstances life has presented you? Sounds ludicrous, doesn't it? Why would anyone ever accept their child has a health issue that can be corrected and not do anything about it?

Accept autism. Do not accept an unhealthy child. Do something

2

about it, and reap the benefits.

The difference between a health problem you know and recognise, and the health challenges outlined in this book, is that the ones I'll discuss later are often hidden. Both will undermine your child's health. If you knew about the hidden issues, I'm sure you would do your best to look for solutions.

Here is the problem: most parents don't know the information you will learn. They remain helpless while their children suffer needlessly. They don't know that they should be investigating underlying health problems, that it's possible to improve many of them, and that doing so can provide tremendous benefits for their children.

My hope is this book changes that for you and for as many other families as possible.

So, how do you approach the information in this book? Think of it as a mission or a quest. You were blessed with a beautiful little human. But now, he or she may have some hidden impediments to their health that are contributing to less-than-optimal wellbeing. Your job is to figure out what they are and address them, so your precious gift can live their life unhindered.

What This Book Offers

At the very core, my goal is to teach you how to get your child as healthy as possible using the following:

- A healthy diet
- Smart supplementation
- Reduction of toxic exposures
- Improved sleep
- Lab testing to identify imbalances and healing opportunities

Sounds simple, yet it's extremely effective when done right. There are many intricacies involved, but by the end of the book, you will understand how to design and implement a customised health-building program for your child. You will do this by:

- Reducing inflammatory foods and harmful food additives
- Minimising exposure to toxic heavy metals and chemicals
- Identifying and addressing gut infections
- Identifying other metabolic imbalances

- Supporting the body's detoxification systems
- Supplementing vital nutrients
- Improving your child's sleep hygiene and environment

To get there, though, I must equip you with the tools and knowledge you'll need but weren't taught.

We also need to clear up a few misconceptions along the way.

It's Not "Because of the Autism"

I want you to understand this because it's critical: nothing that happens to your child, health-wise, is "because of the autism". ASD is a label for a constellation of symptoms, mostly behavioural and highly variable.

An autism diagnosis doesn't "cause" anything. How can this label cause gut dysfunction? How would a diagnosis cause nutrient deficiencies? Or lack of sleep? Can a label cause diminished detoxification capacities and increased toxic burden? The answer is, of course, no. What is more likely is that these health problems are contributing to the autism symptoms and, in some cases, even intensifying them.

Many parents and physicians explain away all kinds of symptoms and behaviours in autistic children as a result of the "autism", when often they are influenced by the health issues listed at the start. And too many doctors still do nothing because they are unaware that they need to look for, and do something about, those imbalances. They just lump all manner of problems under the "because of the autism" umbrella.

Comorbidity is the co-occurrence of two or more conditions in the same person. Among sleep problems, gastrointestinal issues, and immune dysregulation, some of the most common comorbid conditions with ASD include:[23-25]

- Epilepsy
- ADHD (attention deficit hyperactivity disorder)
- Social anxiety disorder
- Specific phobia
- Oppositional defiant disorder
- Obsessive compulsive disorder
- Major depressive disorder

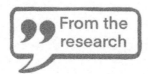

From the research

"Various types of anxiety are believed to be so common in autism that symptoms of anxiety disorders have been thought by some clinicians and investigators to be aspects of autism, rather than comorbid features. Impairing anxiety is, however, not a defining feature of autism or a universal phenomenon of autism. Reported rates of at least one anxiety disorders in individuals with autism have varied from 17% to 84%"[25]

Where does that leave you? Parents are left to struggle on their own, searching for answers. Look at how many books on Amazon focus on "coping" with your child having autism. I'm not disparaging the amazing authors that wrote those books. I applaud them. We need their work. My problem is - where are all the books by authors translating the work of the brilliant researchers working hard to help us understand the physiological mechanisms underlying ASD? No, we don't have all the answers yet. But there is so much valuable information out there. Why is all their research collecting the proverbial digital dust, while kids around the world are suffering needlessly?

This needs to change.

Don't get me wrong, I'm well aware that there are many researchers and practitioners doing incredible work in this area and spreading the vital knowledge needed to help autistic children. But it's not enough. Not nearly enough. One look at the various Facebook support groups for parents is sufficient evidence to confirm this. They just don't know most of the information we'll cover in the coming chapters. It's painful for me to see, though it surely doesn't compare to the pain they are going through.

I didn't want to write this book - I *had* to write it. I couldn't stand idly by while countless kids around the world are suffering from a myriad of maladies that are often relatively easy to identify and address. I felt a sense of responsibility to share this information with you and I'm glad it is in your hands.

So, if it's not the ASD diagnosis causing your child's health issues, what is? I'll be discussing some major culprits in Part One.

Will This Book Complement Other Therapies?

The topics I cover in this book will fit perfectly with other therapies and interventions you may be pursuing for your child, including ones aimed at behaviour. Why? Because if you improve the hardware, the software will function better. Allow me to illustrate what I mean by this.

Think about the following analogy: autism is most often diagnosed by observing a child's behaviour. That's their "software", if you will. But that behaviour largely results from the many underlying physical imbalances in their body, or their "hardware". (Of course, the older a person gets, the more "hard-wired" the behaviour becomes.)

Now think about your phone for a second. The device is the hardware, and the apps on it are the software. If you drop the phone, stamp on it, and spill your tea on it, would you expect it to function well? Probably not.

Likewise, if your child has gut infections, nutrient deficiencies, immune dysfunction, and other "hardware" issues, would you expect their software to work optimally?

In this book, we'll focus on improving your youngster's physical health, the hardware. But, because the software is inextricably linked to the hardware, you may see some improvements in sleep, anxiety, irritability, or other behaviours. You can consider any such improvements a welcome bonus.

Why is My Doctor Not Doing This Already?

You may wonder, "Why doesn't my doctor already address the health issues you mentioned at the outset?" It's not anyone's fault, as such. We're not trying to play the blame game here. Unfortunately, scientific research is slow to reach your doctor. Too slow. In fact:

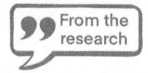

From the research

"It is frequently stated that it takes an average of 17 years for research evidence to reach clinical practice."[26]

It's estimated that it takes an average of 17 years for your doctor down the street to start applying research evidence in their clinic. Surprised? I sure was when I found out. It makes sense when you think about it. First off, it takes time to plan research, apply for and get the funding, conduct the research, and analyse the data. Then you need to write, edit, review, and submit the paper, after which you need to wait for the journal to accept and publish it. Oh, and then you have the small matter of busy physicians having the time to read the paper and decide whether to try out whatever test, intervention, or recommendations were discussed in it.

That's a simplified example, but can you see why this is such a lengthy process? Of course, if you're lucky enough to have a doctor who keeps abreast of the scientific literature, that's great news.

In the meantime, you have the power to take some responsibility into your own hands. I'm not saying you need to read hundreds of research papers. That's why I wrote this book - to save you all that work. But I'm pretty sure you're not prepared to wait 17 years for your doctor to catch up on the scientific literature.

This may seem daunting, but please don't worry. I'm certain that you will soon sense a feeling of empowerment as you process the information in this book and start applying it.

How to Use This Book

Autism is a complex condition, and every case is unique. Just like you don't fix your car or carry out your own dental work, likewise you can't go on this journey alone.

I will educate you, but you must continue to work with knowledgeable clinicians such as your doctor or functional practitioner, nutritionist or dietitian, behavioural specialist, and other experts advising you. You can think of your role as that of a coordinator or project manager, and this book as your guide, but you still need a team of professionals to help you reach your goals.

The *Autism Wellbeing Plan* is divided into two parts. In Part One, I go over the most common health challenges your child is likely to experience, and we lay the foundations for Part Two, where you will put everything you learn into practice.

I recommend that you first read the book from start to finish. Each chapter builds on the previous one and you need these foundations before you begin your child's health-building program. Why? Because if I laid out the wellbeing plan without explaining the reasoning behind it, would you follow it? My guess is many would give up when it gets challenging. But if you know *why* you're doing the things you're doing, you're much more likely to follow through because you understand there is solid science backing your decisions and actions.

Once you've read the book and have started your child's health-building program, you can skip around the sections to refresh your knowledge as needed.

Let me address something important here. I understand that some parts of the book may be a bit dense or technical (especially in Part One). But I beg you, please bear with me through them. I've done my best to only include the most relevant points that you need (this book easily could have been twice as long).

But we can only simplify important information to a point. If you find a section too technical, skip over it and come back another day. This is not the kind of book that you read-through once and cast aside. Nor is it one that you can consume in one sitting. Keep coming back. Your understanding will evolve over time and things will make much more sense.

I promise.

Please don't get discouraged. Power through. Your child will thank you for doing this.

Here is the path you will take to create your *Autism Wellbeing Plan*.

Part One - Health Challenges in ASD

In Part One, I will lay out the foundations you need to fully understand the importance of the recommendations in Part Two.

Chapter One will cover some basics. We begin with an overview of the gut and the role it plays in health. Then, we'll take a brief look at research that has found associations between gut dysfunction and autism severity, as well as anxiety, irritability and challenging behaviours. You'll also learn a few common terms and concepts used throughout the book.

Chapter Two focuses on the immune system. You will get an understanding of the many ways it can go haywire and how this can affect your child's health. We will expand your knowledge of the gut and the role it can play in dysregulating the immune system.

In **Chapter Three**, we discuss gut infections. This is a big piece of the puzzle and an area in which you need to get up-to-speed as a matter of priority. We'll look at how harmful bacteria and yeast can sabotage your child's wellbeing. You will get an overview of some specific organisms that are frequently implicated in ASD, as well as others you might encounter.

Chapter Four covers common nutritional and metabolic imbalances autistic children experience. The more of these you can identify and address, the better off your youngster will be in the long-term.

In **Chapter Five**, we look at how heavy metals, food additives, and other chemicals can undermine your child's health. You will learn about the importance of cleaning up your home to reduce the onslaught of toxins from our modern industrialised environment.

Part Two - Your Autism Wellbeing Plan

After we've laid the foundations, Part Two is where we get into your Autism Wellbeing Plan.

Chapter Six is all about lab testing. You can apply much of the information in this book without running any tests, but there are several that would greatly enhance the effectiveness of the program. I'll discuss testing for gut bugs, nutrient status, heavy metals, and food sensitivities. We'll also get into more specialised tests available to you and the situations in which you might run them.

In **Chapter Seven**, we focus on the healthy gluten-free, casein-free diet and its role in your child's health-building program. I'll clear up some misconceptions about the diet and show you the many benefits it can provide. We'll also briefly review several more advanced diets and the scenarios in which you may need to use them.

Chapter Eight covers the practical aspects of cleaning up your child's diet and environment. By now, you will understand how essential this is. I'll go over the importance of an all-organic diet and some strategies to reduce toxic exposures in your home.

Chapter Nine focuses on improving your child's sleep environment and sleep hygiene.

In **Chapter Ten**, I'll show you the core five supplements you can use to support your child nutritionally.

Chapter Eleven covers more advanced supplementation strategies. We'll look at some of the most useful supplements you can use to enhance your child's health-building program, and the specific situations in which they may be utilised.

Finally, in **Chapter Twelve** is where we put everything you've learnt together. I will show you how to approach the design of a health-building program for your child and give you an example of one. We will consider different scenarios and what to do, depending on your unique situation and test results.

Using the Online Resources

Like I said earlier, this book could have been twice as long. But I had to save you the pain. That is why you will find many more resources on the webpage I built especially for Autism Wellbeing Plan readers: **https://christianyordanov.com/autism-wellbeing-plan-resources/**
There, you will find articles, videos, links to books and further reading, details on lab tests, and all other useful information and updates.

I would also highly encourage you to join my mailing list there. Not only will I send you any future articles, videos, research or other discoveries, I also have a little bonus for you.

When you sign up to the mailing list, I'll send you a link to a free video course on selecting quality supplements for your child. I know many parents are often overwhelmed when it comes to researching and choosing the right supplements. It can be a time-consuming process, but you can take advantage of my extensive research in this area. I will teach you how to avoid junk ingredients, discern between high and low quality products, and evade manufacturers' marketing hype.

Additionally, I'll give you my email address at the end of the book. Please send me your comments and feedback, as well as any questions that arise while you read it. I'll do my best to reply to all emails, and will take your feedback into consideration when preparing updates for the Autism Wellbeing Plan and creating future educational content. If you help me to help you, I will send you a complimentary print copy of the next edition of the book when it's ready.

Getting Started

I hope you're as excited about learning and applying the knowledge contained in this book as I am in offering it to you. I'm confident that if you do your best to implement the core recommendations that follow, you will reap many benefits in the years to come.

Are you ready to begin this wonderful journey of improving your child's wellbeing and your family's quality of life?

Let's begin...

PART ONE - HEALTH CHALLENGES IN ASD

CHAPTER ONE: KEY CONCEPTS

Overview of This Chapter

In this chapter, we'll lay some groundwork. We'll begin by looking at what is required for optimal health and the factors that can diminish it.

We'll then move onto an overview of the gut. You'll learn a lot about this subject in the book because it is so central to your child's health. I'll give you a summary of the research into gut dysfunction and autism severity, and we'll look at how gut issues can contribute to irritability, anxiety, and emotional outbursts. We'll end the chapter by defining some common terms used throughout the *Autism Wellbeing Plan*.

Components of Health

When we talk about physiological health, the following are the most crucial aspects that you need to get right for your child to thrive:

- Nutritious diet, free from harmful chemicals and additives
- A healthy gut
- Restorative sleep
- Exposure to sunshine and nature
- Proper nasal breathing
- Play and movement
- Minimum psychological stress and lots of love and support

If any of the above are out of alignment, your child's health can suffer. You need to do everything within your power to improve each of these factors.

It's clear by buying this book that you have the love and support part already handled. My hope is that by applying what you learn in the *Autism Wellbeing Plan*, you will make great strides in not only improving your child's physical wellbeing but also your whole family's quality of life.

Contributors to Poor Health

There are countless ways poor health can be expressed in the body. Think of how many different ailments, disorders, diseases, and conditions we have classified. Thousands - and we keep coming up with new ones. But there are only a few ways of getting into those states.

Yes, our genes play a role, but even conditions we once thought to be determined solely by genetics are increasingly understood to have a strong environmental influence, including ASD.

An environmental influence can be any factor inside the body or external to it, such as where we live, the food we eat, and exposures to various harmful substances or organisms.

These factors affect how our genes are activated and expressed. What does that mean? It means that while we can't control what genes we inherit, we can exert significant influence over our environment. So, by extension, we exert enormous influence on our state of health (or ill-health). In fact, virtually every single decision we make moves us in one of two directions. On one side is vitality and resilience. On the other is dysfunction, disease, and suffering.

This is a hard pill to swallow for many people because it puts responsibility for their (and their family's) wellbeing directly into their own hands. But I hope you will see it differently. Knowing this information gives you control. It gives you power. You can bring about amazing improvements in your child's health. All that's left is to equip you with the tools you need on your journey.

The primary contributors to diminished health are:

- Low-quality diet
- Nutrient deficiencies or imbalances
- Nutritional excesses (e.g. too much sugar)
- Gut dysfunction

- Pathogenic infections
- Heavy metals and toxic chemicals
- Metabolic imbalances
- Lack of activity
- Poor sleep
- Disordered breathing
- Psychological stress

Of all the above, by far the biggest impact on your child's health is the food they eat. As you will see later, their diet can be a source of nourishment or a source of toxicity.

The Gut's Role in Health

If you forced me tell you what the single most important area you need to focus on improving is - it would be your child's gut function. I know this isn't controversial or ground-breaking knowledge anymore, but I had to write this book because too many parents are still unaware of this crucial information. Meanwhile, their kids are suffering needlessly.

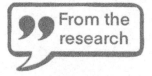

From the research

"Gut microbes are part of the unconscious system regulating behavior. Recent investigations indicate that these microbes majorly impact on cognitive function and fundamental behavior patterns, such as social interaction and stress management. In the absence of microbes, underlying neurochemistry is profoundly altered. Studies of gut microbes may play an important role in advancing understanding of disorders of cognitive functioning and social interaction, such as autism."[1]

What the research is telling us it that, gastrointestinal health affects the whole body. Problems in the gut can cause a myriad of issues elsewhere, not just physical but also behavioural or neurological symptoms, and this is especially relevant in the case of autistic children.

We'll be discussing gut health and how it can affect your child in more depth over the next few chapters. But first, let's have a basic overview of the gut, in case you need a refresher.

Overview of the Gut

When I say gut, gastrointestinal or GI tract, I'll be referring to your child's digestive system. Starting at the mouth and ending at the anus, it includes the stomach, small and large intestines, pancreas, liver, and gallbladder.

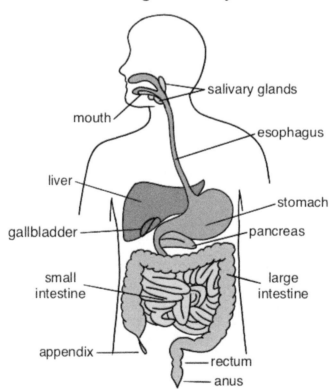

Human Digestive System

Briefly, the major functions of the organs of the GI system are:

- **The stomach** releases digestive enzymes that break down food and acid that kills harmful bacteria.
- **The pancreas** releases digestive enzymes that help to break down food.
- **The liver and gallbladder** release bile that helps with digestion of fats.
- **The small intestine** is where about 90% of nutrients are absorbed. Most of them go to the liver for further processing.
- **The liver** detoxifies harmful substances and processes digested protein and carbohydrates, then sends them out to where they're needed in the body.
- **The large intestine** (or colon) is where the stool is formed, and certain bacteria help to process indigestible fibres and create beneficial compounds such as vitamins and short-chain fatty acids.

Intestinal Barrier

We refer here to the lining of the gut (also known as the mucosal layer or gut barrier). The lining of the intestines is only one cell thick - an unimaginably thin layer. This barrier has the job of keeping toxins and foreign invaders out, while allowing life-sustaining nutrients to pass through into the bloodstream. The intestinal cells also secrete enzymes that help to digest food particles before being absorbed.

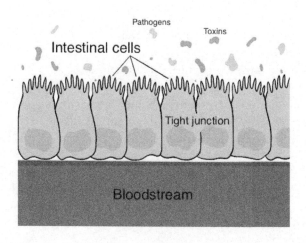

Microbiota

When I use the term gut microbiota, I'll be referring to the community of microbes in your child's gastrointestinal tract. Up to 100 trillion of some 500-1000 species can live in the gut of a human, most of them in the large intestine.[2] Bacteria make up the majority of our microbiota, with some archaea, protozoa, fungi, and viruses making up a much smaller part.[1]

What influences the composition of your child's microbiota? It is now thought that some bacteria begin to colonise the baby while still in the womb. The mother's microbiota, mode of delivery (vaginal or C-section), and the hospital environment dictate to a large degree what microbes will colonise the baby during and after birth. This colonisation plays a fundamental role in brain development early in life.[1]

A child's early microbiota is rather dynamic - many factors can influence and alter its composition, including diet, sleep, medications, toxins, and various other stressors.[3][4]. It is particularly vulnerable to external insults such as antibiotics or toxic substances.

Around two-and-a-half to three years of age, the microbiota begins to stabilise and resemble that of an adult's.[5] After about three years, a child's microbiota becomes much more resilient to change. So if its development was disrupted before that, it may be difficult to balance it, or keep it balanced.

Function of Our Microbiota

We can consider the microbiota as an organ in its own right. The micro-organisms in our gut have a variety of functions and provide many benefits to us, such as:[1][6]

- Helping with nutrient absorption
- Maintaining the gut barrier
- Keeping harmful bacteria in check
- Producing vitamins and other beneficial substances
- Producing neurotransmitters and other similar molecules
- Detoxification of potentially harmful substances
- Regulating the immune system

The microbiota exerts a wide range of effects on our metabolic function[3][7] and expression of our genes.[8][9] Because of the influence it has on the brain, it plays a vital role in behavioural development.[10]

Another amazing thing about the gut is that roughly 70% of the immune cells within the body are located there.[11] The implications of this are that if a child's microbiota is disrupted during critical periods of development, it can have a negative impact on their immune system.[12] As we will discuss in greater depth in the next chapter, a disrupted immune system can lead to all manner of health problems.

The Gut-Brain Axis

We used to think our brain was the command centre of the body, sending out signals to control our organs' functions. But more recently, we've discovered that the microbes in our gut can produce molecules that can influence the brain, and by extension how we think, feel, and act.[1]

The gut and the brain have a two-way communication system which keeps them informed about each other via a complex network of pathways that include our hormones, immune and nervous systems, and molecules that our microbiota produce.[13]

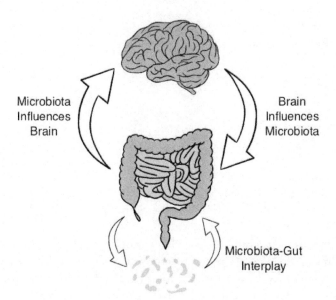

Gut-Brain Axis

Microbiota Influences Brain

Brain Influences Microbiota

Microbiota-Gut Interplay

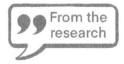

"Although the exact etiology and pathology of ASD remain unclear, a disorder of the microbiota-gut-brain axis is emerging as a prominent factor in the generation of autistic behaviors."[14]

Let me translate the above quote: although we don't yet know the exact causes or ways in which ASD develops, a disruption of the communication pathways between the gut microbiota and the brain are now thought to be a significant contributor to autistic behaviours.

In simpler terms, your child's gut can influence their mind, mood, and behaviour by affecting or regulating:[12][14][15][16][17]

- Appetite and satiety (the feeling of fullness after a meal)
- Emotions and attitude
- Learning and memory
- Stress response and anxiety
- Response to pain

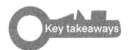

To sum up what we covered so far, your child's microbiota is influenced by diet, sleep, medications, toxins, and other stressors. The microbiota influences the brain and your child's "software".

Are you starting to see the connection here? Yes, your child's diet, sleep quality, exposure to toxins or antibiotics, and stress levels will exert direct and indirect influence on their behaviour, focus, intellectual functions, emotions, and all the other software. In large part, this will be due to the effects these factors have on their microbiota. What we're talking about here is of huge importance.

Here is the critical piece of the puzzle: we have a lot of scientific research showing that the gut microbiota is often disrupted in autistic children.[18-23] We'll be discussing the implications of this (and what you can do about it) in much of the rest of the book.

What is a Healthy Gut?

To be considered in a healthy state, your child's gut needs to be able to:[24]

- Break down, extract, and absorb nutrients from food
- Provide nutrients and energy to the body's organ systems
- Identify what it should allow into the body and what it should not
- Keep out foreign substances and maintain the integrity of the gut barrier
- Maintain the beneficial bacteria and eliminate harmful organisms

If any of these functions are not working properly, the subsequent imbalances can cause your child many health complications.

Gut Dysfunction and How it Can Affect Your Child

I'll be using the terms "ASD severity" or "autism severity" quite a lot, so let me briefly explain what that will mean in this book.

You may already know that there are numerous rating scales, checklists, and questionnaires used to help diagnose autism. Commonly used ones include:

- CARS (Childhood Autism Rating Scale)
- ADOS (Autism Diagnostic Observation Schedule)
- ADI-R (Autism Diagnostic Interview - Revised)
- ATEC (Autism Treatment Evaluation Checklist)
- GARS-2 (Gilliam Autism Rating Scale, 2nd Edition)
- ABC (Autism Behaviour Checklist)

Each assessment method is different, but the end result is usually a score or rating that can be used to determine how severe the autism diagnosis is. (I realise that these tools are crude and using labels like mildly autistic or severely autistic is not at all liked in the autism community, and I fully agree. Using these labels can be perceived to either minimise the challenges the individuals face or their abilities. But such are the limitations of science, so I hope you won't be put off by these terms.)

ASD researchers use some of the above tools in their studies. They may evaluate the children using one or more rating scale, then measure certain physiological markers of interest to them in that particular study. For example, they may measure heavy metals in blood or hair, or assess the gut microbiota of the study participants. After collecting the data, they analyse it and look for correlations or associations.

Let's say, after crunching the numbers, the study participants with more severe autism tended to have higher levels of heavy metals than those with low or moderate scores. Then the researchers will report that heavy metals were associated with higher autism severity.

Now you know what I mean when I say a factor has been associated or correlated with ASD severity. If it's not completely clear yet, we will look at some examples shortly that will help to clarify.

Where am I going with this? It's now well established in the scientific community that gastrointestinal problems are common in autistic children[25] and that they may exert an influence on autism severity.[26-29]

The research we have so far has shown that anywhere from 9% to 91% of ASD study participants had at least one gastrointestinal problem.[30-33] The most common symptoms reported are:

- Constipation
- Diarrhoea
- Reflux
- Abdominal pain
- Bloating
- Excessive gas, burping, or belching

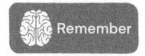
Remember

Now, please understand: the above symptoms are outward manifestations of *underlying issues*. Why is that important to know?

Simple. If you and your practitioner can figure out what the underlying causes are and address them, then the outward gut symptoms are much more likely to improve, or even go away.

Only treating the symptoms is a terrible strategy. It's like spray-painting the leaves of a tree green when they wilt and turn yellow, instead of watering it and adding fertiliser to the soil. I know it's a ridiculous analogy, but the current paradigm of treating only symptoms without looking deeper is just as ridiculous and is doomed to fail.

Some of the most common underlying causes or contributors to GI symptoms include:

- Poor diet
- Intestinal permeability (leaky gut)
- Gut infections (parasites, bacteria, fungi)
- Food allergies or sensitivities
- Inflammation
- Impaired digestion, digestive enzyme deficiencies
- Immune system irregularities

Okay, what's the good news? The positive news is that you can do something to improve all of the above factors. That's what the *Autism Wellbeing Plan* will teach you.

Gut Issues and Autism Severity

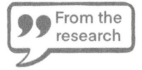

From the research

"The strong correlation of gastrointestinal symptoms with autism severity indicates that children with more severe autism are likely to have more severe gastrointestinal symptoms and vice versa. It is possible that autism symptoms are exacerbated or even partially due to the underlying gastrointestinal problems."[27]

Several studies have analysed the association between gastrointestinal problems and autism severity.[26-28] One study reported that, when compared to autistic children without GI problems, those children *with* gut issues showed greater symptom severity on measures of irritability, anxiety, and social withdrawal.[26]

Another paper reported that autistic children with gut problems had worse scores on the ATEC subscales of speech, social, sensory cognitive, and health and physical behaviour.[27]

Similarly, another study found that autistic children were more likely than typically developing peers to have at least one frequent GI symptom. Of the autistic group in the study, they found that those with more frequent abdominal pain, gaseousness, diarrhoea, constipation, or pain when pooping, scored worse on irritability, social withdrawal, stereotypy, and hyperactivity when compared with children having no frequent GI symptoms.[28]

Of course, just because two things are correlated (gut dysfunction and autism severity), it does not necessarily mean that one is causing the other.

However, one study found that treatment with the antibiotic vancomycin (which only works in the gut) was effective in reducing autistic symptoms temporarily.[29] This suggests that gut dysfunction (in this study, likely a bacterial infection) does play a role in causing (or increasing) autistic symptoms.

When considering the results of the above studies along with others we'll look at later, we can build a strong case that gut dysfunction can indeed contribute to behaviours or symptoms generally considered as "autistic".

By the end of the book, you will know how to investigate and address various GI problems your child may have. The result will be a healthier child and a happier you.

Gut Issues, Anxiety, and Challenging Behaviours

When you think about it, it's only logical that constipation, diarrhoea, abdominal pain, and bloating can worsen a child's symptoms or behaviour.

Tummy trouble can make anyone cranky, so it should be no surprise that if your child has gut issues, they will be more irritable, or will act out in other ways.

Sometimes, gut dysfunction can lead to more serious things like self-injurious behaviour and even aggression towards others. These issues can become even more pronounced if your child has communication difficulties or is non-verbal, because they won't be able to express their discomfort to you.

Challenging behaviours are one of the most significant factors influencing your, and your child's, quality of life. That is why it's important to get a grip on as many of the physiological factors contributing to them. If you can do that, behavioural strategies and interventions will have a higher likelihood of being effective.

Like I've said, if you improve the hardware, the software can run more smoothly.

Research has shown that autistic children can express gastrointestinal symptoms in emotional and behavioural ways, including:[34][35]

- Irritability
- Agitation
- Aggression
- Noncompliance to requests
- Self-injurious behaviour
- Tics

There are studies showing that autistic children who also had gut conditions tended to be more anxious[36] and irritable[37] than children without GI problems. Another study found that children with gut dysfunction were more likely to display oppositional defiant behaviours and tantrums than children without GI issues.[38]

Of course, any child (even without gut complaints) may show these behaviours, so the behaviours in and of themselves won't always mean there's an underlying GI issue. But it's a good idea to keep this information at the back of your mind next time you notice irritability, aggression, or emotional outbursts. They could be a clue that your child has discomfort they can't express.

In Chapter Twelve, I'll show you some more subtle clues that your child may have hidden gastrointestinal issues. We'll now look at some ways in which the gut can become dysfunctional.

Intestinal Permeability (Leaky Gut)

Intestinal permeability, or "leaky gut", is a state where the spaces between the cells of the gut increase. Thus, the intestinal barrier becomes more *permeable*.

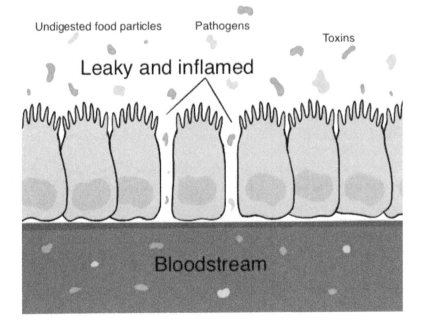

These gaps allow undigested bits of food, bacterial toxins, and other particles that shouldn't be there to enter your child's bloodstream. Once there, the immune system perceives these particles as foreign invaders, so it revs up and starts attacking them. What happens next is a cascade of inflammation and immune reactions that can lead to:

- Food sensitivities
- Food maldigestion and malabsorption
- Damage to the intestinal lining and further permeability
- Toxins and bacterial metabolites may enter the bloodstream
- Autoimmunity

What Can Cause Leaky Gut?

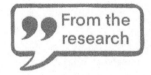

"Toxic chemicals such as mercury, aluminum, formaldehyde, glutaraldehyde, bisphenol-A, artificial food coloring, in the environment and in food products, and vaccines or medications, have the capacity to break the oral tolerance mechanism and increase intestinal permeability."[39]

Many factors can contribute to leaky gut. The most common are:[39-41][42]

- Inflammation
- Gut infections
- Food allergies or sensitivities
- Heavy metals and chemicals
- Gluten
- Food additives
- Physical and emotional stress

Prevalence of Leaky Gut in ASD

ASD researchers have found increased intestinal permeability in 26% to 76% of their study participants.[43-47] Interestingly, a study that found that 37% of the autistic patients had abnormally high intestinal permeability, also found it in 21% of their first-degree relatives. In contrast, less than 5% of the control group participants had excessive intestinal permeability present.[43] This could mean there are familial factors at play that predispose the members of the same family to increased intestinal permeability.

What's also worth mentioning here, is that the autistic individuals in that study who were on special protein-restricting diets (e.g. wheat and dairy free), had significantly lower intestinal permeability than those not on such diets.[43]

We'll cover diet later in the book, but I hope I just planted a seed in your head about the potential benefits of the gluten-free, casein-free diet. There are many misconceptions out there about it and I hope we can clear them up for you as you continue reading.

Gut Pathogens

Pathogens, or gut bugs, are harmful organisms that can proliferate in your child's gut and cause serious health problems. The most common types of pathogenic organisms are:

- Parasites
- Bacteria
- Fungi (yeasts and mould)
- Viruses

When pathogenic organisms invade the gut, we call this a state of "dysbiosis".

What is Gut Dysbiosis?

Dysbiosis is a state of imbalance in the gut. It is a broad term that can mean any combination of the following has occurred:

- The good bacteria have decreased in numbers
- Opportunistic or pathogenic organisms have overgrown or invaded your child's gut
- Your child's digestive function may be impaired (e.g. poor digestion or absorption, low stomach acid or bile production, digestive enzyme deficiencies, altered intestinal motility)

Now that we've covered the importance of the gut in health, I probably won't need to work as hard to convince you that dysbiosis is one of the most important concerns to address when striving to improve your child's health.

Many factors can contribute to dysbiosis, including:

- Decreases in the good bacteria
- Pathogenic infections or overgrowths
- Leaky gut and other digestive dysfunction
- Poor diet
- Food sensitivities
- Immune dysfunction
- Toxin exposure (heavy metals, chemicals such as pesticides)
- Medications (antibiotics, antacids, anti-inflammatories)

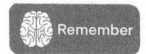

Please remember this: your child may not have apparent gut symptoms, but this does not automatically rule out gut dysbiosis. As I mentioned earlier, many seemingly uncon-nected issues, including behavioural changes or even skin problems, can stem from underlying gut dysfunction.

Key Takeaways

To wrap up our whirlwind tour of the gut, here's a summary of the key points I need you to keep in mind as you progress through the *Autism Wellbeing Plan*:

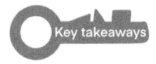
Key takeaways

- The intestinal barrier is only one cell thick.
- The microbiota's composition is influenced by diet, sleep, medications, toxins, and other stressors.
- Our gut microbes influence our mood, behaviour, and brain function.
- Various factors can contribute to leaky gut and dysbiosis, including inflammation, infections, food allergies or sensitivities, heavy metals, and chemicals.
- Problems in the gut can manifest elsewhere in the body, as physical, behavioural, or neurological symptoms.
- A child's microbiota stabilises around three years of age, making it much more resilient to changes. Prior to that, it is particularly vulnerable to various toxins and other stressors.
- Research has shown autistic children to have a high prevalence of gut issues and disrupted gut microbiota.
- Gut dysfunction has been associated with autism severity, anxiety, irritability, and certain challenging behaviours.

We will develop your understanding of how leaky gut and dysbiosis can undermine your child's health in the coming chapters.

Important Terms and Concepts

Before we wrap up this chapter, I need to introduce you to a few terms I'll be using throughout the rest of the book.

Don't worry about understanding them in great detail. For now, I just want you to have a conceptual understanding that we can build on as you progress through Part One.

Inflammation

Inflammation is a protective process that the body initiates when it is injured in some way. That's known as *acute* inflammation and it's healthy - but it should be temporary.

The problem with many health challenges experienced by autistic kids is that they cause *chronic* inflammation, which is disease-promoting. We'll discuss the plethora of ways inflammation is caused in the body in various parts of the book. We'll also consider strategies to lower it and keep it as low as possible in Part Two.

Oxidative Stress

Oxidants, or free radicals, as they're sometimes called, do the opposite of what antioxidants do in the body - they cause damage, rather than protect against it. Oxidants are highly reactive, unstable atoms or molecules that can injure cell membranes, proteins, DNA, and other important biochemical structures.

Oxidative stress is a process where the body's antioxidant protection is not enough to prevent damage from free radicals and other oxidation reactions. While negative factors can cause production of oxidants, they are also a natural by-product of our metabolism that the body can normally keep in balance. It is when the body's antioxidant defence systems are overwhelmed or depleted that we have a problem.

Factors that cause or contribute to oxidative stress include:[48]

- Heavy metals and toxic chemicals
- Depletion of the body's antioxidants such as glutathione (see next section)
- Certain medications
- Gut infections

Aside from damaging important proteins and structures, oxidative stress can induce inflammation and cause premature death of our cells, mutations in our DNA, and can even be cancer-promoting.

Brain cells are especially vulnerable to oxidative stress because their membranes are made from polyunsaturated fatty acids that oxidise easily. Because brain cells do not replicate, once damaged, they may become permanently dysfunctional or may die and never be replaced.

Researchers have documented oxidative damage or markers of increased oxidative stress in autistic individuals in numerous studies.[50-53] It appears that, for various reasons we'll discuss later, autistic children are more susceptible to increased oxidative stress. We'll examine common contributors to this detrimental process and things you can do to reduce it in your child.

Glutathione

Glutathione is the most powerful antioxidant our bodies make. It basically plays a role in protecting us from all sorts of harmful things - from toxic metals and chemicals, to infections and oxidative stress.

Low levels of glutathione are common in autistic children, as has been evidenced by many researchers.[49-62] Its levels can get depleted when there is a lot of oxidative stress in the body (which you now know is common in autistic children).

Depletion of glutathione can lead to:

- Reduced ability to detoxify heavy metals and chemicals
- Impaired immunity
- Increased oxidative stress
- Impaired DNA synthesis and repair

We'll discuss strategies to support your child's glutathione production and to reduce the stressors that deplete it in Part Two of the *Autism Wellbeing Plan*.

Methylation

Methylation is the addition of a single carbon and three hydrogen atoms (known as a methyl group) to another molecule. It is an important biochemical process that happens countless times in the body every second and has roles in:

- The immune system

- DNA expression
- Energy production
- Detoxification of heavy metals and chemicals
- Hormone and neurotransmitter metabolism
- Many other vital functions

A shortage of methyl groups can impair some of these processes, which can lead to a negative chain of events in the body. Many nutrients, genes, and enzymes are involved in the methylation cycle, which means many things can go wrong with it.

A large body of evidence has shown that autistic children have significantly impaired methylation.[51][54][55][61-63]

Toxins

I'll use the terms "toxin" or "toxic compound" when referring to anything that can be harmful to the body. The most common categories of toxins we'll focus on in this book are:

- Heavy metals (e.g. mercury, lead, aluminium, arsenic, cadmium)
- Chemicals (e.g. BPA, phthalates, pesticides, food additives)
- Bacterial and fungal by-products and metabolites

Neurotransmitter

When you see terms that start with "neuro", we're talking about something related to the brain and nervous system.

A neuron is a nerve cell - they're found in the brain and nervous system. They help us perceive our environment and operate our bodies, both consciously and unconsciously.

Neurodevelopment is the development of the brain and nervous system - obviously an extremely important process for a growing child.

Neurotransmitters are chemicals our neurons use to communicate with each other. Many are derived from amino acids (the building blocks of proteins) and even some basic amino acids themselves can serve as neurotransmitters (e.g. glycine and glutamate).

A neurotoxin is any compound that is harmful to our neurons. Neurodegeneration is a process where the neurons lose their structure and functions over time (which may include the death of the neuron).

Blood-Brain Barrier

The blood-brain barrier can be compromised by many factors, particularly by a leaky gut combined with circulating bacterial toxins and chemicals or heavy metals. When disrupted, it can lead to damage or dysfunction of neurons, and even neurodegeneration.[50][64]

A child's blood-brain barrier is not completely formed until around six months after birth, which makes babies especially vulnerable to toxic exposures.[65]

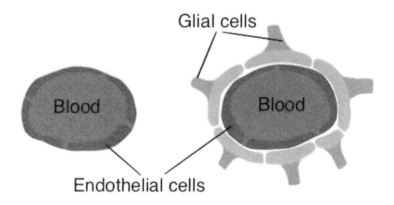

Mitochondrial Dysfunction

Mitochondria are the tiny organelles in our cells whose primary role is to produce energy. They do this by burning glucose and fatty acids to produce ATP, which is the molecule we use to "carry" energy in the body. You may remember mitochondria from biology class as the "powerhouses of our cells".

Our mitochondria are remarkably sensitive to various stressors, and when they are dysfunctional in any way, it can affect our energy levels, gut function, and even our brain and muscles. We will tackle this important topic in more depth in Chapter Four.

Wrap-up

In this chapter, we laid the foundations for the rest of the book. We looked at the core pillars of health and the factors that can contribute to diminished wellbeing.

I took you on a quick tour of the gut and you saw how imbalances located there can manifest elsewhere in the body, not just physically but also as behavioural or neurological symptoms. We took a brief look at some research showing that gut dysfunction has been associated with autism severity, anxiety, irritability, and certain challenging behaviours. You also learnt some key terms and concepts that we will develop over the upcoming chapters. Again, I just introduced you to them and you don't need to worry about understanding them in great depth - things will start making more sense as you keep reading.

Now it's time to get a better grasp of the major contributors to poor health that can affect autistic children.

In the next chapter, we'll look at the topic of immune system dysregulation. You will learn about factors that can disturb a child's immune system, and we will further expand our discussion of the role the gut can play in causing ill-health when dysfunctional.

CHAPTER TWO: IMMUNE SYSTEM DYSREGU-LATION IN ASD

Overview of This Chapter

In this chapter, I will introduce you to some terms related to the immune system, then we'll look at ways in which it can get dysregulated. We'll pay particular attention to the role the gut can play in this.

Why are we starting with this topic? The reason is that abnormalities in the immune system are very common in autistic children.[1-5] These can manifest as an over-active immune system or other imbalances, such as the elevation of inflammatory molecules (e.g. cytokines) and lower levels of anti-inflammatory or regulatory immune molecules.[3][6]

Many studies have found associations between blood markers of immune activation and inflammation, and the severity of certain behaviours in ASD. In other words, when certain immune molecules were elevated or too low, the children had higher scores on the behavioural measures used to determine ASD severity.[2][7-9]

Examples of behavioural associations with dysregulated immune system markers included:[2][7-9]

- More impaired social behaviours and communication
- Increased restricted, repetitive, and stereotyped patterns of behaviour and interests
- Lower adaptive behaviours and worse behavioural symptoms

- Poor social development
- Increased irritability, hyperactivity, or lethargy

Please keep in mind that this topic is vast. Though a lot of research has been done already, much more is needed to elucidate fully the various mechanisms that can cause immune dysfunction in ASD.

While we'll only scratch the surface here, it should be enough to give you an idea of the many things that can go wrong with a child's developing immune system, and some effects it can have. After a brief review, we'll look at what you can do to positively influence your child's immune system.

First, let's define a few terms we'll be using.

Terms Related to the Immune System

Innate and Adaptive Immunity

The immune system protects us from pathogens. It monitors our internal environment and responds swiftly to all potentially harmful attackers. You can think of the immune system as having two departments: the innate arm and the adaptive arm.

We are born with the innate immune system. Through it, our bodies can sense micro-organisms and compounds that need to be neutralised, broken down, or excreted from the body. An immune response from the innate arm is sometimes also referred to as a cell-mediated immune response.

The adaptive arm, as the name implies, is "trained" as we get exposed to new bacteria, viruses, and other organisms throughout our lives. An immune response from the adaptive arm is also called a humoral immune response.

What can happen if one of the departments is out of sync with the other?

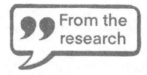

"Together these immune responses function as a harmonious symphonic orchestra. When disharmony occurs or the tempo loses the beat, the immune dysfunction, due to elevated inflammatory cytokines and down-regulation of regulatory cytokines, may contribute to ASD."[6]

Basically, if the two arms of the immune system are not working in proper coordination with each other, inflammatory molecules (cytokines) may start getting produced in excess, while anti-inflammatory ones won't be produced in sufficient amounts. Imbalances like this can lead to health issues over time.

Immune Dysregulation

When the immune system is functioning properly, it protects us from pathogens and does not react to the foods we eat or attack our beneficial bacteria. But when it is constantly activated or imbalanced in other ways, we start to have problems like chronic inflammation or autoimmunity.

Because such a large part of the immune system is found in the gut (about 70% of it), an imbalance there can cause a cascade of negative reactions in your child's body. Remember, these reactions won't necessarily be physical - they can manifest as mood, behavioural, or cognitive disturbances.

Antigen

An antigen is anything that the immune system may perceive as a foreign invader that it must eliminate. It can be a part of an infectious organism, a heavy metal or chemical, and even a food particle under certain circumstances.

Antibody

When the immune system determines something is an antigen, it tags it and starts producing antibodies (also known as immunoglobulins) that will recognise and attack it.

Antibodies are produced by the adaptive arm of the immune system. Each one is created specifically for every new antigen that enters the body.

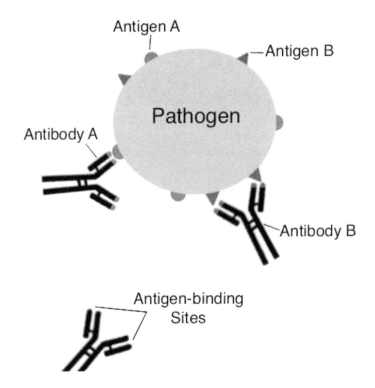

Autoantibodies and Autoimmunity

For various reasons we'll discuss later, the immune system may some-times mistake the body's own tissues as antigens that need to be at-tacked. That's when autoantibodies are created that can target parts of the person's cells, proteins, or other self-tissues. We call that autoim-munity. Autoantibodies are one of the main mechanisms of autoim-mune disorders.

How Does the Immune System Get Dysregulated?

Many factors can lead to immune dysregulation. In one study, the authors stated:

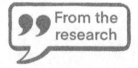

"The question remains - what is causing the chronic immune activation of the brain? We believe that there is compelling evidence that excessive systemic immune stimulation through a combination of numerous and closely spaced vaccinations, immune and excitotoxic effects of the mercury additive thimerosal, systemic infections, food allergies, Candida infections, and genetic factors all play a part."[10]

Basically, any number of internal or external stressors can perturb the immune system of a growing child, from infections and allergies, to toxins in food or medications. Some individuals may have a greater genetic susceptibility, which can make them more vulnerable to these stressors.

In this section we will take a closer look at the following common contributors to immune dysfunction:[1]

- Maternal factors
- Allergies
- Autoimmunity to self-proteins
- Activation of microglia
- Inflammation caused by the innate immune system
- Heavy metals and toxic chemicals
- Gut infections and leaky gut

Maternal Factors

Researchers are increasingly finding links between maternal autoimmunity and autism. For example, disorders such as autoimmune hypothyroidism, rheumatoid arthritis, type I diabetes, and psoriasis have been associated with a higher incidence of ASD when the mother has them during pregnancy.[1]

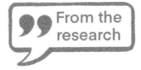

From the research

"In summary, the results of these familial studies do not single out one autoimmune disease and risk for ASD; however, a clear familial autoimmune component has emerged. The significant overlap of autoimmunity within the family members of ASD subjects may suggest an involvement of inherited immune factors. Maternal autoimmunity could also be playing a role in the gestational immune environment that has been found to significantly influence neurodevelopment."[1]

Other than autoimmunity, common maternal factors that can dysregulate the development of the child's immune system include:[1]

- **Gestational immune activation** such as viral or bacterial infections.
- **Compromised microbiota** of the mother during pregnancy.
- **Autoantibodies**: researchers have identified autoantibodies that can react with the brain tissue of the growing foetus in some mothers of autistic children.
- **Maternal allergies** can also play a role.

Now, maternal factors such as the above are clearly outside your control but I included this discussion for the sake of completeness. You need to be aware that certain influences over the immune system's development cannot be modified.

But many can be modified, so we can't dwell on what we can't control. This is a wellbeing plan for the now and the future. All we can do is strive to do our best with the tools and resources we have. Part Two of the book will ensure you have as many tools in your arsenal as possible.

Allergies

Researchers are showing that there is a higher prevalence of allergies in autistic individuals.[1]These include asthma, hay-fever (allergic rhinitis), and eczema (atopic dermatitis).

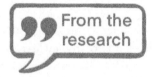

From the research

"Practicing physicians should be aware of the potential impact of allergic diseases on behavioral symptoms and cognitive activity in ASD children."[11]

An allergy is a hypersensitivity disorder of the immune system. Dysregulation in both innate and adaptive immunity can contribute to the development of allergic diseases.[12]

One large study found that asthma was 35% more common in children with autism than their peers.[13] Another one found a higher risk of developing asthma and other allergic disorders in autistic individuals.[12]

In some cases, allergies may influence ASD severity and some core behaviours. Researchers have found children with more severe autism to have a higher prevalence of allergic disorders.[14]

Another paper I read reported that autistic children not only had more allergies than neurotypical controls, but the autistic children who had gut issues had more allergic disorders than those without gut symptoms. The researchers also noted that autism severity was associated with higher blood IgE levels (which are markers for allergies). Simply put, children with higher allergic markers tended to have more severe ASD symptoms.[15]

Because allergies can cause stress, pain, discomfort, and sleep deprivation, they can also contribute to irritability, hyperactivity, and otherwise aggravate the behavioural symptoms in autistic children.[11]

Unfortunately, allergic disorders may go undetected for a long time and cause many kids extra unneeded and preventable suffering, as one paper noted:

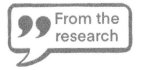
From the research

"It has been our experience that in ASD children, behavioral changes caused by both IgE- and non-IgE-mediated diseases are often attributed to just being 'autistic' and no proper diagnosis and treatment for the child's condition was implemented prior to their arrival at our facility. Our observation indicates the need for physicians involved in the care of ASD children to be aware of the importance of diagnosing common allergic as well as nonallergic diseases in these children. It is also important for the physician to not attribute certain symptoms displayed by ASD children to just being 'autistic', even if the symptoms are frequently associated with ASD."[11]

Autoimmunity to Self-Proteins

Studies have found autistic subjects to have various antibodies in their blood to "self-proteins" such as those of the gut barrier, brain, and central nervous system tissues, as well as other cellular components.[1][16-19]

Autoantibodies like these are a common feature of autoimmunity, and their presence may be predictive of the development of certain autoimmune conditions.[1] Like many disorders, autoimmunity is a spectrum, so autoantibodies may also be present in healthy people and it won't always mean the person will develop an autoimmune disease.

However, researchers have found levels of antibodies to cerebellar neurons (brain cells) to be associated with ASD severity.[19] In that study, children with more severe autism had higher levels of antibodies than children with mild-to-moderate autism (measured with CARS). Other studies have also found ASD severity to be associated with antibodies to tissues in the brain.[20]

Given that antibodies to brain cells and other structures in the central nervous system directly bind with those tissues and damage them, it makes sense that higher levels of antibodies were correlated with more severe manifestations of autism.

Causes of Autoimmunity

But what causes these antibodies to get produced in the first place? It's a complex question with no straight answer. There are many pathways to autoimmunity in the body and every person's unique genetic makeup and environment influences their susceptibility. However, we do know some possible mechanisms that may play a role.

Cross Reactivity / Molecular Mimicry

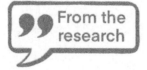

From the research

"Due to the similarity of food proteins and infectious antigens to human tissues, antibodies produced against the food and infectious antigens may also attack human tissues."[21]

A cross-reaction is said to happen when an antibody for an antigen also reacts with one of our own tissues (which could be a part of our brain, gut barrier, or anything else). This can happen when the antigen and our tissue share similar structures.

Basically, the antibody is roaming around in the blood looking for the bad guy (antigen) to attack. But it sees our own tissue first and mistakes it for the antigen because they resemble each other. This process can quickly turn into a vicious cycle where more antibodies are produced that further damage our body's tissues.[21]

Cross Reactivity

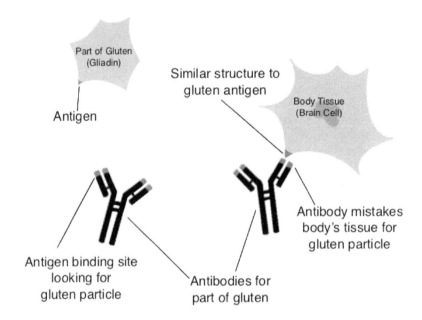

Possible cross-reacting antigens include:[19][21][22]

- Food allergens (e.g. soy, wheat, or cow's milk proteins)
- Heavy metals (e.g. mercury)
- Chemicals or their metabolites
- Infectious agents (e.g. bacterial toxins, *Candida albicans*, viruses)

Formation of Neo-Antigens

Some heavy metals, chemicals or their metabolites, and even food particles can bind with our own tissues. In effect, they get "stuck" in them, forming a new structure or "complex", called a neo-antigen.[21]

This process makes it more likely that our body will attack our own tissue because when the immune system doesn't recognise the neo-antigen, it can react strongly against it.[21]

That's not all, though:

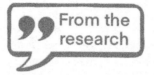

"The act of binding to tissue also breaks down tissue, causing tissue antigens to free-flow through the bloodstream. Here the immune system will identify these tissue antigens as unwanted materials, and thus make antibodies against them. Once the formation of autoantibodies occurs, tissue degeneration may follow. This is autoimmune reactivity. If the exposure to the environmental trigger is not eliminated, the tissue destruction will continue to the point of autoimmune disease."[21]

To put it in simpler terms, the very act of compounds binding to our tissues damages them and causes them to break down. Pieces of our own tissues can get into the bloodstream, where our immune system marks them as antigens. Can you see how this can quickly escalate? Now the immune system is producing more antibodies to structures that resemble parts of the body. Over time, this process of autoimmune reactivity causes damage to those tissues. Worse yet, if it occurs in the brain or nervous system, it can result in neurodegeneration and contribute to loss of brain function.

Compounds that can bind with human tissue include:[6][21]

- Chemicals and heavy metals (e.g. mercury, aluminium, BPA, formaldehyde, artificial food colourants)
- Dietary lectins and agglutinins (e.g. parts of gluten)

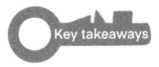

What's the key takeaway here? You need to identify and eliminate as many potential triggers that can either cross-react or
form neo-antigens in your child's body as possible.

Activation of Microglia

Glial cells (plural: glia) are found in our central nervous system. Some
key roles they play there include protecting neurons structurally and
from pathogens, and supplying them with nutrients.

Microglia are one type of glial cell that has been shown to play a role
in ASD. They are the resident immune cells within the brain and central nervous system. Microglia are normally in a resting state, but certain things can activate them. When they are activated, they secrete
compounds that can be neurotoxic, including inflammatory molecules,
glutamate, and quinolinic acid (these last two are powerful excitotoxins, a concept we'll discuss in Chapter Four).[23]

Some activation of microglia is required for neurodevelopment, but
chronic activation (as is the case for many autistic children) can cause
neuroinflammation and neurodegeneration.[1][10]

Factors that can activate the microglia include:[23][24]

- Aluminium
- Mercury
- Dietary excitotoxins (e.g. MSG)
- Certain pesticides
- Systemic immune activation
- Infections (bacterial, viral, fungal)
- Food allergies

Inflammation Caused by the Innate Immune System

When the innate immune system is overactive or dysregulated for any
reason, it can cause complications in the body that can contribute to

poor health. The inflammation that accompanies innate immune acti-vation can cause over-activation of the adaptive arm which can lead to prolonged illnesses, reactions to foods or compounds which weren't a problem before, and to autoimmunity.[1][25]

You might be wondering, what causes the inflammation in the first place? As you'll discover over the course of reading this book, many factors can cause or contribute to it, including gut infections, toxic sub-stances, and food sensitivities.

Heavy Metals and Toxic Chemicals

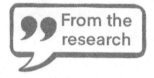

"Environmental pollutants such as heavy metals, solvents, and pesticides have been shown to dysregulate the immune system potentially resulting in immune suppression, auto-im-mune conditions and/or hypersensitivity states."[26]

A significant, though often ignored, contributor to immune dysfunc-tion is toxic exposure. It is so significant that we have a whole chapter on the topic (Chapter Five), and another section that addresses how to reduce your child's exposure to the countless toxic chemicals and heavy metals in our environment and food supply (Chapter Eight).

Gut Infections and Leaky Gut

Much research has already shown that the gut microbiota strongly in-fluences the immune system and plays a major role in its dysregulation in ASD.

Our gut microbiota not only regulates the immune system of the intestines, but can exert great influence on the entire body, directly and indirectly, via many complex mechanisms.[27]

It goes even beyond the fact that 70% of the immune cells within the body are located in the gut.[28] The microbiota actually shapes the innate and adaptive arms of the immune system. By that I mean that our im-mune cells are "trained" or "educated", of sorts, in the gut. After this, they can take part in immune processes throughout the body.[29]

What are the implications of this? They are far reaching, because exposure to different bacteria causes the formation of specific types of immune cells - some of which are protective, while others can be damaging.

Depending on what's going on in the body, the microbiota may cause the immune system to produce inflammatory or anti-inflammatory compounds. These molecules can then influence brain function, cause or reduce inflammation elsewhere in the body, and affect a myriad of other processes.[27]

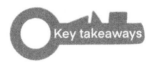

Key takeaways

In other words, when we have harmful bacteria running rampant and causing dysbiosis in the gut, it will lead to systemic effects that will most likely be inflammatory and activate the immune system.

We will address the topic of gut infections and dysbiosis in much more depth in the next chapter. Let's now examine how a leaky gut can contribute to immune dysfunction.

Leaky Gut and Inflammation

We discussed leaky gut and factors that can worsen it in the last chapter. You know that food allergies or sensitivities, pathogens, heavy metals, and toxic chemicals can increase intestinal permeability. With it, inflammation is a common occurrence that can cause:[30]

- Damage to the intestinal cells and further intestinal permeability
- Reduced digestive capacity due to decreased enzyme secretion
- Impaired absorption of nutrients

Impaired digestion and absorption increase the risk of nutrient deficiencies or inadequacy, which can lead to many negative knock-on effects in the body. But that's not all:

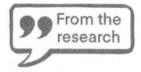

"Due to low activity of digestive enzymes in ASD patients, food antigens from different sources may survive as intact proteins or peptides, and the immune reaction against them may result in antibody production against the food proteins or peptides. If there is antigenic similarity between the food protein or peptide and human tissue structures, the food antibodies may cross-react with tissue antigens. The end result could be autoimmune reactivity followed by autoimmune disease."[6]

Once the intestinal barrier is breached and becomes leaky, this allows partially undigested food particles, heavy metals and chemicals, and bacterial toxins to get into the bloodstream more easily.[31] Once in there, the result is further immune activation and inflammation that can lead to autoimmunity.

Are you starting to see how a damaged gut can cause all manner of health issues?

It is a vicious cycle that will self-perpetuate unless you take action to arrest the process.

From Leaky Gut to Leaky Brain

Our potential problems do not end there. Because the gut and brain are tightly connected and regulated by each other, dysfunction in one will invariably affect the other.

To recap, here is the scenario we have so far:

- The gut barrier is breached and becomes "leaky"
- Undigested food particles, heavy metals, chemicals, and bacterial toxins get into the bloodstream
- The immune system is activated, resulting in inflammation and production of antibodies

What can happen next? As you know from the first chapter, the blood-brain barrier is there to protect the brain and nervous system. But once a leaky gut allows various toxins to circulate in the blood, they can inflame and damage the blood-brain barrier, and eventually cause it to open up.[32] We call this increased blood-brain barrier permeability, or "leaky brain" for short.

Another key thing to note is that the blood-brain barrier is made of some proteins that are also present in the gut barrier. As the gut is damaged, some of those proteins can break off and end up in the bloodstream. When that happens, the immune system marks them as antigens (they shouldn't be there) and starts producing antibodies against them. Those circulating antibodies can now attack the blood-brain barrier.[21]

Do you see where I'm going with this? Once the blood-brain barrier gets disrupted, the circulating pathogens, metals, chemicals, and the antibodies to them can get inside the brain and nervous system. There, they can wreak havoc and exert negative effects on behaviour.[21]

This has been confirmed by researchers who have found antibodies to blood-brain barrier proteins (and other brain tissues, as we covered earlier) to be significantly higher in autistic children than in their peers.[6]

Neuroinflammation and Neuroautoimmunity

Once the blood-brain barrier gets breached, inflammation and autoimmunity of the brain and nervous system become possible.

The processes that cause neuroautoimmunity are similar to those that cause autoimmunity in the rest of the body, which we covered earlier. To briefly sum them up, they are:[32]

- **Inflammation** in the brain and central nervous system, caused by various assaults, including pathogens and toxins.
- **Cross-reactivity (or molecular mimicry).** Antibodies created for environmental toxins, gluten, casein, or pathogens mistake brain or nervous system tissues for those antigens.
- **Formation of neo-antigens.** Chemicals, metals, or food particles (e.g. lectins or agglutinins) can bind to brain or nervous system tissues. This process can damage the affected tissues and cause the immune system to react to them.

When the immune system targets neurological tissues, the resulting damage can manifest as behavioural problems, movement disorders, and communication difficulties.[32] Over time, this can lead to neuro-degeneration and negative effects on cognition, development, and many other physiological processes.

I'll leave you with this quote from a research paper before we look at some things you can do:

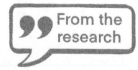

"The earlier the environmental triggers are detected and re-moved, the better will be the clinical conditions of ASD pa-tients."[21]

What Can You Do About It?

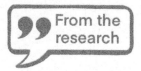

"While a panacea for such a heterogeneous disorder may never exist, evidence suggests that manipulation of the immune re-sponse could improve core features of ASD as well as associ-ated aberrant behaviors."[7]

You might wonder, what are some indications that your child's im-mune system is dysregulated? Common physical clues include:[33]

- Food allergies or sensitivities
- Obvious adverse reactions to foods, chemicals, or medications
- Chronic gastrointestinal symptoms (e.g. constipation, diar-rhoea, excessive gas, bloating)
- Recurrent infections not responding to the first-line treatment (e.g. ear infections, chronic sinusitis)

If your child exhibits any of the above, it means that deeper investigation is warranted on the part of your health care provider. Below are some things you can do to positively influence your child's immune system. We'll be discussing these topics in more depth in the coming chapters.

- Identify allergies and eliminate allergens from the diet and environment (some children may benefit from immunotherapy)
- Identify food sensitivities and remove reactive foods from the diet (Chapter Six)
- Remove other potentially cross-reactive or inflammatory foods and additives (Chapter Seven and Eight)
- Clean up your child's environment to reduce exposures that can activate or dysregulate the immune system (Chapter Eight)
- Identify and address gut infections that are causing immune activation (Chapter Three, Six, Eleven, and Twelve)
- Support gut healing with a healthy organic diet and supplements (Chapter Seven, Eight, Ten, and Eleven)
- In some cases, you may want to test for autoimmune antibodies (Chapter Six)

We will review the above in Chapter Twelve, where we put everything you've learnt together.

Wrap-up

As you saw, many elements can conspire to disturb your child's immune system and undermine their wellbeing. From maternal influences during pregnancy, allergies, and microglial activation, to inflammation, toxins, and gut dysfunction.

While you cannot exert control over all of them, many are within your sphere of influence. The challenge is to figure out what the dominant factors are in your child's unique case and set of circumstances, and address them.

Thankfully, we have a lot of tools at our disposal. The best part is, you'll be able to start applying some of them immediately.

Now that you have an overview of the many ways the immune system can get dysregulated, it's time to focus in on a major one: the dreaded gut bugs.

CHAPTER THREE: GUT INFECTIONS AND DYSBIOSIS - A BIG PIECE OF THE PUZZLE

Overview of This Chapter

In this chapter, I'll show you how pathogenic infections can sabotage your child's health. We'll take a closer look at a few specific organisms such as the *Clostridia* family of bacteria and the infamous yeast *Candida*, because they are often implicated in ASD. I'll also give you a quick primer on mould, which is an emerging area of interest in ASD research.

Given how much research has been done in this area, it's still shocking to me how many parents still are unaware of how common gut infections and overgrowths are in autistic kids - and that there's a great deal they can do about them.

Numerous studies have found imbalances and disruption in the gut composition of autistic children.[1-11] Most often observed are reductions of important beneficial bacteria (e.g. *Bifidobacteria* and *Lactobacillus* species) and overgrowth of certain species that are considered pathogenic.[12][13]

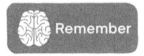

Please keep in mind that while I'll cover a few pathogens in this chapter, there are dozens of common ones that may be causing your child distress. From parasites and protozoa, to opportunistic bacteria and fungi.

This is why you'll hear me stress the importance of testing for gut bugs throughout the book. It's probably the most important test to run because addressing different types of pathogens requires different approaches. Most importantly, unless you get rid of the bad bugs, you can't expect your child to reach optimal health.

How Gut Infections Contribute to Poor Health

Gut infections have been implicated as a causal factor in many conditions, including allergic, autoimmune, and inflammatory diseases. Always remember that your child will not necessarily present with gastrointestinal symptoms if they have an underlying infection.

Pathogenic infections in the gut can:

- Damage the intestinal lining and increase leaky gut
- Promote inflammation
- Contribute to immune dysfunction and promote autoimmunity
- Keep the body in a state of chronic stress (which can contribute to other disorders)
- Increase oxidative stress levels
- Produce a variety of harmful by-products
- Contribute to decreased beneficial bacteria
- Cause malnutrition or nutrient deficiencies
- Increase food sensitivities
- Contribute to liver congestion and dysfunction
- Create an environment conducive to proliferation of secondary overgrowths, biofilm, and further infestation

Different organisms produce various metabolic by-products by feeding on the carbohydrates and protein that your child eats. While some are beneficial, others can be harmful. The state of your child's microbiota largely determines which direction it goes.

If beneficial bacteria (e.g. *Bifidobacteria* and *Lactobacillus*) numbers are high, and pathogens are low, most of the bacterial by-products will nourish the intestinal lining, regulate the immune system, and otherwise keep your child's gut healthy (and by extension, other systems of the body will function well).

However, if there is dysbiosis in the gut - let's say there is a bacterial infection, yeast overgrowth, and beneficial bacteria levels are low - then there will be much higher production of harmful by-products. When you add to this leaky gut, nutrient deficiencies, or other metabolic imbalances, you have a recipe for poor health.

Unfortunately, many autistic children live like that for years.

If you find your child is in that state, you need to work to reverse the process in the other direction. More on that later, first let's see how the substances our microbiota produce can affect us.

Short Chain Fatty Acids' Role in Health

Our gut bacteria can digest and ferment sugars and complex carbohydrates (e.g. dietary fibre) in the large intestine to produce short-chain fatty acids (SCFAs) such as butyrate, acetate, and propionate. These can affect not only the gut barrier's stability but can also exert effects on the brain and nervous system. This is, in part, because due to their size and structure, SCFAs have the ability to cross the gut barrier and get into the bloodstream, while some may even get through the blood-brain barrier.[14]

The levels of SCFAs produced are largely determined by the composition of our microbiota. Like all other things in the body, we need a certain balance for optimal health.

For example, butyrate-producing bacteria play a vital role in maintaining the intestinal barrier because butyrate is the preferred food for cells in the large intestine. When butyrate-producing bacteria's numbers are reduced due to dysbiosis, it can affect the integrity of the gut barrier and disrupt the immune system of the gut (which will have profound systemic effects).

Dysbiosis leading to a reduction of butyrate can result in:[14]

- Impaired intestinal barrier function

59

- Inflammation
- Bacterial toxins or metabolites entering the bloodstream (causing immune activation or directly influencing the brain)
- Other dysregulation of the metabolism

Likewise, *too much* of certain SCFAs can cause imbalances in the body. One of these that has received a lot of attention in the scientific community is propionate.

Propionate's Implications in ASD

Propionate, also called propionic acid, is produced by many bacteria, including *Clostridia, Desulfovibrio,* and *Bacteroidetes.*[14][15]

Some of these propionate-producers are pathogenic and have been shown to be elevated in autistic children. (We'll discuss *Clostridia* and *Desulfovibrio* shortly.)

While normal levels of propionate are thought to be beneficial, too much of it can have negative effects on health and behaviour.[16] Though much more research needs to be done so we can better understand the mechanisms, we have accumulating evidence supporting the hypothesis that propionate contributes to ASD. In a nutshell, the main points are:[15-18]

- Propionate concentrations are often higher in autistic children than their peers in studies.
- Autistic children treated with antibiotics that target propionate-producing bacteria show temporary improvement in autism symptoms.
- People with impairments in propionate metabolism exhibit neurodevelopmental conditions with behavioural and biochemical similarities to ASD.
- Animal studies have shown that propionate can induce autistic-like behaviour and other neurocognitive impairments, as well as inflammation, oxidative stress, and glutathione depletion. All of these are characteristic of ASD.
- Propionate disrupts carnitine metabolism in animal studies and carnitine imbalances have been found in autistic children. (More about carnitine in the next chapter.)
- Antibiotics (beta lactams) commonly used for routine infections in children alter the gut microbiota in favour of propionate-producing bacteria. Beta lactams can also impair carnitine metabolism directly.

Propionate can exert negative effects on:[16][19][20]

- Gastrointestinal function
- Mitochondrial function and energy production
- Immune function
- Communication between cells
- Gene expression
- Neurotransmitter synthesis and release
- Fatty acid metabolism

Bacteria aren't the only source of propionate. It is used as an anti-fungal preservative in a variety of foods, including refined wheat and dairy products, and is naturally present in some foods such as cheese.[16][19][20] It can also be produced in the body under certain circumstances, however, bacteria such as *Clostridia* are the most significant source of propionate for a large majority of autistic children.

Lipopolysaccharides and Bacterial Toxins

Lipopolysaccharides (LPSs) are fragments of bacterial cell walls. They are powerful immune system activators, capable of inciting inflammation in the body.[22][23] LPSs and other bacterial toxins (called endotoxins) play a role in many disorders of the gut, liver, immune and hormone systems.[15][23]

LPSs and other endotoxins can open up the gut barrier and eventually get into the bloodstream. Once in our systemic circulation, they can target the blood-brain barrier and also cause it to start opening up. Once they penetrate the brain, LPSs can trigger neuroinflammation, seizures, and autoimmunity.[15][24]

As you learnt in the previous chapter, a leaky blood-brain barrier will also allow other molecules in that shouldn't be there, such as heavy metals, pathogens, and circulating antibodies.[23]

Biofilm

Some pathogenic organisms can organise themselves into what we call biofilm communities. Examples of biofilms include the plaque that forms on our teeth and the slime-like formations often found in damp areas around the home. These communities can form not only in our digestive tracts, but in other cavities, such as the sinuses.

Biofilms are surprisingly resilient and sophisticated structures. Bacteria and yeast use them to protect themselves, to take in nutrients and pump out waste, and as a communication network. Once hidden in biofilm, pathogens become much harder to get rid of. They can evade the immune system and antibiotics, and cause serious health issues for the infected person.

Bacteria

Let us now take a closer look at two families of bacteria that have been implicated in ASD, *Clostridia* and *Desulfovibrio*.

Clostridia

The Clostridia family of bacteria have been receiving quite a lot of attention in the scientific community with regard to ASD. Most Clostridia species seem to be non-pathogenic commensals (i.e. beneficial or at least not harmful to us),[25][26] however a few of them can be particularly harmful.

Several studies have found increased or abnormal numbers of Clostridia species in the guts of autistic children.[3][27][28] One of those studies found that gastrointestinal complaints in autistic children were significantly associated with Clostridia bacteria.[28]

Perhaps the most well-known of the pathogenic members of the family is Clostridium difficile. It can cause serious illness and kills tens of thousands of people each year. Other harmful members include Clostridium tetani, Clostridium perfringens, and Clostridium botulinum.

Many Clostridia species are resistant to a lot of antibiotics, including common ones used to treat ear infections. In part, this is because some species are spore-forming. The spores are resistant to heat and antibiotics,[29] which makes them difficult to eliminate. They can survive our stomach acid and other defence mechanisms.[30] Thus, antibiotic treatment could leave behind harmful Clostridia or their spores while wiping out our protective beneficial bacteria, leaving us vulnerable to dysbiosis.

An important study in the early 2000s found that autistic children not only had more Clostridia species (and in higher numbers) than their peers, but also that the autistic children had spore-forming species whereas the neurotypical controls didn't have any at all.[27]

Spores can survive outside the body and many regular household disinfectants (such as alcohol wipes) only spread them.[30] Bleach kills spores, but it is too harsh of a cleaning product to use regularly, especially around youngsters. This poses a risk because Clostridia spores can lay dormant for long periods of time and can begin proliferating only when the person's microbiota gets disrupted (e.g. by antibiotics).[31]

Urinary Metabolites of *Clostridia*

Clostridia are highly metabolically active. They can ferment carbohydrates and some amino acids (building blocks of protein) to produce a range of compounds that can be toxic to the gut, brain, and nervous system. One of them is propionate, as we just covered. But there a couple others we need to talk about.

Why do we need to go in such depth, you wonder? The main reason is that we have the means to measure certain *Clostridia* metabolites in urine, using organic acids testing. This means we can detect the presence of *Clostridia* bacteria and do something about them. This is probably one of the most important things I will teach you.

We will talk about the organic acids test a lot in this book because it is so valuable to run on autistic kids, beyond just detecting pathogens and dysbiosis. If you're eager to read up about it, please see Chapter Six, where I cover the most important lab tests you can run.

We'll now take a glance at the following compounds:

- 4-cresol (also called p-cresol)
- HPHPA (3-(3-hydroxy phenyl)-3-hydroxypropionic acid)

Don't worry too much about remembering their names for now. Chapter Twelve will include all the information you'll need. For now, we're just laying the foundations of the knowledge you will need later.

4-cresol (p-cresol)

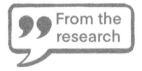

"Potential sources of p-cresol excess in ASD, such as gut infection, chronic constipation, antibiotics, abnormal intestinal permeability, and environmental exposure, are being investigated. P-cresol may contribute to worsen autism severity and gut dysfunction, often present in autistic children. It may also contribute to a multibiomarker diagnostic panel useful in small autistic children."[32]

Clostridium difficile has the ability to ferment the amino acid tyrosine,[33] with 4-cresol (also called p-cresol) being the main by-product from this process.

There are other sources of p-cresol, including certain foods, cosmetics, household products, and from the environment. However, it is bacteria that seem to exert the greatest influence on the production of this compound and others related to it.[32]

What's so bad about it? 4-cresol inactivates the enzyme dopamine-beta-hydroxylase (DBH), which converts the neurotransmitter dopamine to noradrenaline (norepinephrine, if you're in the US).[34] This reaction is irreversible because the 4-cresol gets stuck in the enzyme, rendering it permanently inactive. When the DBH enzyme is inhibited, dopamine can build up in the brain and central nervous system. At the same time, not enough noradrenaline is produced, leading to an imbalance of these important neurotransmitters.

Why is too much dopamine bad? For starters, dopamine is a very reactive molecule. Even when it is degraded as part of our natural metabolism, it produces by-products that can damage structures around it. An excess of dopamine can lead to:

- Damage to neurons due to oxidative reactions
- Depletion of the antioxidant glutathione in the brain and nerve cells (which makes them more vulnerable to oxidative stress and toxic chemicals or metals)

- Imbalances in the nervous system

Here's where the organic acids test comes in handy. Not only can we measure 4-cresol with it, but it also has markers for dopamine. So, we can detect *Clostridium difficile* and see if there are neurotransmitter imbalances.

Some more reasons why you would want to detect 4-cresol and address the *Clostridia* overgrowth:

- 4-cresol is toxic to other bacteria in the gut, including other Clostridia species. This means that elevations of this compound in the gut can have a negative impact on the microbiota.
- Constipation can lead to a build-up of toxins in the gut that can get into the bloodstream, especially when the gut is leaky. One study found that young autistic children with chronic constipation and increased intestinal transit time had elevated levels of 4-cresol.[35] (This is one of the many reasons why you need to keep your child pooping regularly to make sure potential toxins are flushed out of the system before they can cause problems.)
- The same group of researchers found that higher 4-cresol levels were associated with higher autism severity[36] and behavioural abnormalities.[37] These findings further indicate that this metabolite plays a neuroactive role in ASD.

Here is a summary of the key points:

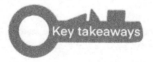

Key takeaways

- 4-cresol has been implicated in ASD and can cause health problems
- We have the means to detect 4-cresol with the organic acids test (discussed in Chapter Six)
- We know what to do about *Clostridium difficile* overgrowth (discussed in Chapter Twelve)

Are you starting to get the picture? You can find out whether *Clostridia* overgrowth is a problem for your child and do something to address it, which will result in improved health.

HPHPA

HPHPA is another chemical that can be detected with the organic acids test. It is often seen in autistic children who have little or no speech, or low muscle tone.

HPHPA is produced by *Clostridium botulinum, Clostridium sporogenes, Clostridium caloritolerans*, and several others.[29] Similar to 4-cresol, this bacterial metabolite can also inhibit the DBH enzyme and cause other neurotransmitter imbalances in the brain.[38]

Desulfovibrio

Researchers have identified species of the *Desulfovibrio* bacteria family in stool specimens of autistic children.[5]

Desulfovibrio are sulphate-reducing bacteria (they "breathe" sulphate instead of oxygen) and may be, in part, to blame for the abnormalities in sulphur metabolism found in many autistic children. (We'll cover sulphation, an important process in the body, in the next chapter.)

One study found *Desulfovibrio* in the stools of 50% of the autistic participants and some of their siblings, but not at all in any of the neurotypical study participants. The researchers noted that the higher counts of *Desulfovibrio* were associated with increased autism severity.[5]

Some ways *Desulfovibrio* can disrupt our health include:[5][39]

- May cause alterations in sulphate metabolism
- They produce LPSs that can get into the bloodstream and aggravate the immune system
- Can slip into protective biofilm to evade antibiotics and the immune system
- Produce propionate
- Produce hydrogen sulphide, a potential mitochondrial toxin, which may act synergistically with propionate to promote mitochondrial dysfunction.

Fungal Infections and Overgrowths

We have a lot of fungi living inside us and they are typically not a threat if we're healthy. It's when our immune system or gut lining get compromised that opportunistic fungal species can proliferate and cause us problems. In this section, we'll discuss two types of fungi that can impair your child's health - yeasts, namely the *Candida* family, and mould.

Candida

Candida species are the dominant yeasts in our digestive tracts. These are tiny, but incredibly sophisticated organisms. When allowed to overgrow, due to dysbiosis or antibiotic use, they can cause us issues in various ways. I'll outline a few of them so you're aware of how *Candida* can undermine your child's health and understand the importance of identifying and addressing yeast overgrowths as soon as possible.

For starters, *Candida* can exist in its single-celled form, but they can also join together into a community where they become more pathogenic. They then start to release root-like structures (called hyphae) that can push through the intestinal lining and increase leaky gut.[15] They also produce various enzymes that can break down the digestive tract.

But we are only getting started here. *Candida* are literally competing with your child for the nutrients he or she eats. They take sugar (glucose) and produce various chemicals that can affect your child's metabolism and mood. Some of these are alcohol and acetaldehyde.

Yes, you read that correctly! Yeasts can produce alcohol through the metabolism of sugar, that's why we use them to make beer and wine. If they can do that in a barrel, why wouldn't they do that in your gut? In fact, *Candida* can contribute to children's giddy or goofy behaviour. They can be, in effect, somewhat "drunk" when *Candida* overgrow and are given plenty of sugar through the diet.

Acetaldehyde is a by-product of the breakdown of alcohol in the liver and contributes to the feeling of a hangover after drinking. *Candida* can produce this chemical through the sugar fermentation process on the way to making alcohol (ethanol). As you can imagine, you don't want this compound circulating in your child's body if you can help it. Acetaldehyde affects the methylation cycle negatively and can disrupt the metabolism of some neurotransmitters such as dopamine.[15]

It doesn't end there. *Candida* produce other chemicals that have similar structure to ones our bodies make. They look similar but disrupt our metabolic processes because they don't behave in the way our bodies would expect.

Other ways in which *Candida* can impair your child's health include:[15][40]

- Affect the immune system and cause the production of inflammatory compounds
- Can metabolise amino acids into ammonia
- Produce gliotoxin, which can damage DNA and is toxic in other ways
- Candida are even known to be able to escape immune cells that have swallowed them and thus gain access to other parts of the body

Candida and other yeasts tend to overgrow in the following scenarios:

- Gut dysbiosis caused by other pathogens
- When the immune system is disrupted
- High-sugar diet
- Antibiotic use or over-use (which kills good bacteria that keep *Candida* numbers in check)

What's the link with autism? Numerous studies have identified *Candida* overgrowth in autistic children using various methodologies.[1][41-46] On the positive side, this is another organism that we can detect with the organic acids test, so we'll be revisiting this topic in Chapter Six and Twelve.

Mould and Mycotoxins

Interest in the role of mould and the toxins they produce (called mycotoxins) in ASD has been growing recently,[47-49] with some evidence emerging that certain mycotoxins may contribute to ASD.[47][48] Even if they don't contribute to autism directly, they can still play a role in diminishing your child's health.

Mycotoxins are some of the most prevalent toxins in our environment. Because they are heat resistant, they contaminate a vast portion of our food supply in the fields, storage, and in processing. We also get exposed to them through inhalation as mould can grow inside buildings, especially those that have been water damaged.

Mycotoxins can contribute to ill-health through various mechanisms, such as:[15][50-53]

- Being toxic to cells (e.g. causing mitochondrial dysfunction)
- Suppressing the immune system, increasing vulnerability to other pathogens
- Toxic to the kidneys, liver, and other organs
- Causing DNA damage (DNA damage caused by mycotoxins has been shown to be carcinogenic)
- Contributing to oxidative stress
- Damaging the gut barrier and increasing intestinal permeability
- Depleting glutathione, leading to impaired detoxification capacity
- Certain species can produce oxalate crystals (see Chapter Four)

The risks with mould are twofold:

- The mycotoxins themselves are harmful
- The fungi can infect and colonise the human host

A Quick Primer on Mould and Mycotoxins

The most common mycotoxins are produced by the fungi families (genera) of *Aspergillus, Fusarium, Penicillium,* and *Stachybotrys.*

- **Aspergillus** is the most prevalent species in the environment. The most common way to get exposed is simply breathing within an indoor environment that has mould growing in it. The *Aspergillus* spores are tiny, which allows them to reach our lower airways. This can lead to fungal colonisation. Some mycotoxins that *Aspergillus* species produce are ochratoxin A and aflatoxins. Ochratoxin A is by far the most common mycotoxin in the environment.
- **Fusarium** grow on various types of grains including corn, wheat, rice, and barley. They produce fumonisins, as well as zearalenone, a mycotoxin that resembles oestrogen, giving it oestrogenic properties (as well as being harmful to the liver, DNA, and immune system).
- **Penicillium** is the blue-green mould that grows on fruits, vegetables, and in indoor environments. They can also contaminate

seeds and grains. *Penicillium* species produce ochratoxin A among other mycotoxins.

- **Stachybotrys** is the greenish-black mould that can grow on drywall (gypsum board), paper, wood composites (fibreboard), and ceiling tiles. They grow in higher humidity environments than other fungi.

Other common mycotoxins, such as patulin and gliotoxin, are produced by multiple moulds, including *Aspergillus* and *Penicillium*.

Patulin is the most common mycotoxin found in apples and pears, and further products derived from these fruits such as juice, compotes, baby food, and other foods intended for young children.[54]

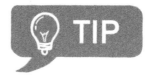

Testing for mycotoxins at the outset of your child's health-building program is not necessary in most cases. In Chapter Twelve, I'll show you the circumstances in which you need to consider it.

Other Pathogens: Parasites and Worms

Before we wrap up our brief review of pathogens that can impair your child's health, I want to remind you that we only scratched the surface.

Parasites are another large category of organism that are always a risk, no matter the age of the person. It is quite easy to get infected, especially for kids that are crawling around on the ground, playing with pets, and putting all sorts of things into their mouths.

Some of most common sources of exposure to parasites are:

- Contaminated water
- Faecal contamination of food and liquids
- Improper hand hygiene
- Contact with infected people or animals

The problem with parasites is that they promote an environment in the gut where harmful bacteria and yeasts thrive. That makes it impossible to get rid of those pathogens and heal the gut fully until the parasites have been addressed.

This is why, as you'll see in Chapter Six, I recommend running both the organic acids test and a comprehensive stool test, if you can. The organic acids test is great at detecting yeast and *Clostridia*, while a quality stool test will detect parasites and other harmful bacterial species.

What Can You Do About It?

In Part Two of the *Autism Wellbeing Plan*, you will learn how to:

- Identify pathogens through urinary organic acids and stool testing (Chapter Six)
- Design a protocol to support pathogen eradication (Chapter Eleven and Twelve) in partnership with your practitioner
- Support your child's gut healing using diet, supplementation, and lifestyle interventions

Wrap-up

In this chapter, we looked at the many ways in which pathogenic organisms can cause our bodies, our "hardware", distress. That in turn can cause our software to have glitches. You learnt some fairly technical details about the various substances the micro-organisms in the gut can produce, and their potential negative effects in the body.

You became acquainted with the bacterial families *Clostridia* and *Desulfovibrio*. I showed you two *Clostridia* metabolites that we can detect using the organic acids test - this will come in handy in Part Two of the book when you start putting everything you've learnt into action.

I also gave you an overview of how fungal infections and overgrowths can contribute to ill-health. You saw how surprisingly sophisticated the tiny *Candida* yeasts are, and some ways in which they can affect your child. We wrapped up that section with an overview of mould and mycotoxins - an often-overlooked source of ailment in some susceptible individuals, and an area which I'm certain will receive a lot more attention in the future.

As you're aware by now, there are many pieces in the puzzle that is your child's journey to better health. With this chapter behind you, it's now time to expand our view from the gut to the broader metabolism. That is the next chapter's focus.

CHAPTER FOUR: COMMON NUTRITIONAL AND METABOLIC IMBALANCES IN ASD

Overview of This Chapter

In this chapter, we'll examine some common nutritional and metabolic challenges autistic kids experience. I'll build the case for why you need a robust supplementation program to support your child, even with a great diet. We'll also take a brief look at what the research into autistic children's diet adequacy has discovered.

The remainder of the chapter will focus on the following:

- Zinc and copper imbalance
- Vitamin D deficiency
- Low omega-3 fatty acids
- Iron deficiency
- Mitochondrial dysfunction
- Carnitine deficiency
- Glutathione status
- Impaired methylation
- Excess glutamate and excitotoxicity
- Sulphate and sulphation impairments
- Elevated oxalate levels

Don't worry if some of the above are unfamiliar to you. By the end of the chapter, you will have a solid understanding of these topics. Also, keep in mind that while we're focusing on a lot of health issues in this part of the book, Part Two is all about working to identify and correct as many of them as possible. So, please don't let the information dampen your spirits. Remember - knowledge is power.

The Importance of Nutrient Supplementation in ASD

There are three main factors that will affect your child's nutritional status:

- **Nutritional**: the diet itself
- **Behavioural**: eating habits and food preferences
- **Physiological**: gut function, food allergies or sensitivities, genetics, metabolic abnormalities, and existing nutrient deficiencies or imbalances

As you can see, optimal nutritional status depends not only on what you feed your child but also on how it's digested, absorbed, and processed in their body. A properly functioning gut is crucial for them to extract the maximum value from their diet.

What does this mean? It means the challenge of improving your child's nutritional status is three-fold: providing the right nutrients, getting them to eat the food, and removing any impediments that can prevent those nutrients from being assimilated.

As you progress through this chapter and the rest of the book, I hope that you will realise that the case for a well-designed, high-quality supplementation program for your child is strong. We'll get into much more detail later, but in a nutshell, the main points are:

- Autistic children are notoriously picky eaters and tend to self-select limited diets[1][2]
- Selective eaters are at an increased risk for many nutrient deficiencies including calcium, zinc, vitamin D, and vitamin B_{12}[3]
- Studies of nutritional intake have found many nutrient inadequacies in autistic children's diets
- Gut dysfunction can hinder proper assimilation of the nutrients your child's diet provides

- Metabolic challenges such as impaired methylation and increased oxidative stress may deplete nutrients or cause imbalances[4]
- Increased toxic burden can also deplete vital nutrients
- Certain mineral deficiencies can increase absorption of some toxic metals[5][6]

Nutritional Inadequacy Heightens Toxicity of Metals

One particularly harmful consequence of nutrient inadequacies is that they can leave your child more susceptible to heavy metal toxicity. Some examples of how this can happen include:[5][6]

- Iron deficiency increases absorption of cadmium, lead, and aluminium
- Calcium deficiency can increase lead absorption
- Zinc deficiency can increase cadmium absorption in the gut
- Deficiencies of calcium, iron, and zinc enhance the negative effects of lead on cognitive and behavioural development
- Selenium protects from mercury toxicity, thus low selenium intake can increase the harmful effects of mercury

We will revisit the topic of how heavy metals sabotage our health in the next chapter.

Research on Food Intake in ASD

Many researchers have looked at autistic children's nutritional intake by surveying their parents. Naturally, when you consider how picky and self-selecting autistic kids can be in terms of their diet, you can imagine that nutrient inadequacies are woefully common.

The most commonly reported nutrients to be insufficient in the diets of autistic children are:[2][7-11]

- Vitamin A
- Vitamin C
- Vitamin D
- Calcium
- Iron

Other nutrients found to be insufficient, in at least one study, include:[2][7-9][11-12]

- Zinc
- Magnesium
- Selenium
- Choline
- Vitamin B_2, B_3, B_5, B_6, B_7, folate and B_{12}
- Vitamin E
- Vitamin K
- Potassium

A study in 2010 reported that some of the autistic children who took part had an inadequate intake of several nutrients including vitamin A, vitamin C, and zinc, but the most common were vitamin D, vitamin E, and calcium. Strikingly, <u>83% of the children had 3 or more nutrient inadequacies</u>. None had zero, which mean every single one of those children in the study had at least one vitamin or mineral inadequacy in their diet.[2]

Overall, the patterns of inadequacy seem to be slightly different across different regions of the world, which is to be expected. Your child's dietary preferences, your shopping habits, the food availability in your region, seasons of the year, and other factors will influence your child's nutrient intake profile.

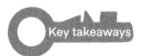
Key takeaways

The key point to take away is this: we cannot immediately assume that your child's diet is inadequate, but we should be compelled to inspect it more closely.

The research certainly supports the case for you to track your child's food intake for at least 3 typical days, preferably even longer. Gathering this data will allow you to do some basic analysis that can identify any serious nutritional gaps in their diet. It doesn't have to be complicated. I'll show you how to track and analyse your child's diet easily in Chapter Twelve.

Nutritional Status: Beyond Vitamins and Minerals

I've read a lot of research on ASD, and while vitamin and mineral inadequacies or deficiencies are common, there are other problems lurking that many doctors and parents miss.

Here is an example. One large comprehensive study found that autistic children, when compared to neurotypical peers, had lower levels of some vitamins and minerals. Not much surprise there. But perhaps even more important is that the researchers also found the autistic children had lower glutathione, increased oxidative stress, and impairments in methylation and sulphation.[4]

As we discussed at the outset of the book, increased oxidative stress, lower glutathione, and impairments in methylation are a common occurrence in autism, and can lead to serious health consequences over time. The study authors wrote:

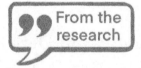

From the research

"An important issue in the clinical care of ASD children is that most vitamins, minerals, and plasma amino acids were within the reference range, but other biomarkers (oxidative stress, methylation, sulphation) were very abnormal, suggesting that those other biomarkers can be important guides for treatment."[4]

What am I getting at here? For starters, to be "within the reference range" on a blood test is no measure of health. Most reference ranges are way too wide and tell us very little. Many labs define their ranges from the entire group of people that they test. Now, who is more likely to get a lab test, a healthy person or an unhealthy person?

My point is that your child's basic blood test results may come back "normal" or within the labs ranges. That does not mean there isn't a deeper metabolic issue that may need to be addressed, and it certainly doesn't mean that the levels are optimal for them.

Here's an example. If your child's zinc is at the bottom of the range and their copper is at the top of the range, your doctor might send you home with nothing to worry about. However, that doesn't mean the zinc and copper are in the right balance and this isn't causing your child problems.

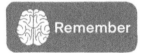

Please remember this as you read on because it's important: "within the lab range" does not mean healthy. Many nutritional and metabolic imbalances are hidden deeper, thus they need better investigation (and more comprehensive programs to address them) on the part of your clinician. Do not settle for less.

Common Imbalances and Deficiencies

Let's review some common nutritional and metabolic imbalances that affect autistic children. This is not going to be an exhaustive list, but it will give you an idea of how many things you could be investigating and addressing. Even identifying and correcting three or four issues could do wonders for your child's health.

Zinc and Copper Imbalance

An imbalance of zinc and copper is one of the most common nutrient imbalances in the general population, and the most common one in ASD.

Low zinc and elevated copper have been found to be a contributing factor to not only autism but also ADHD, insomnia, headaches, fatigue, muscle and joint pain, hypertension, premenstrual syndrome, depression, and many other disorders.[13]

These two minerals need to be maintained in a fairly tight ratio for optimal health, and their imbalance has even been associated with ASD severity. Let's examine them in more depth.

Zinc

After iron, zinc is the most abundant trace mineral in the body and is required for the functioning of hundreds of enzymes. Zinc is found in the brain, muscles, bones, kidneys, liver, and parts of the eyes, and plays important roles in:[13]

- Immune function
- Brain development and functioning
- Neurotransmitter regulation
- Wound healing
- Protein and DNA production
- Cell division and cellular metabolism
- Protecting against oxidative stress
- Supports normal growth and development during pregnancy, childhood and adolescence

Dietary sources of zinc include:[13]

- Beef and lamb
- Cheese
- Liver
- Oysters
- Pumpkin seeds

It's a good idea to think about your child's diet for a moment. If they don't eat much meat, zinc intake is likely to be low.

Zinc Deficiency

Several factors can cause zinc deficiency, such as:

- Inadequate intake
- Malabsorption due to gut issues or anti-nutrients in food (e.g. phytate in grain products)
- Too much copper, which is antagonistic to zinc
- Chronic diarrhoea leads to excessive zinc loss

Zinc deficiency or inadequacy can cause, or is associated, with:[13][14]

- Growth delays
- Impaired immune function and increased risk of infections

- Impaired digestion, malabsorption of food
- Dysregulation of some neurotransmitters
- Impairment of antioxidant defences and increased oxidative stress
- Impaired DNA repair capabilities in the body
- Increases vulnerability to heavy metals
- Delayed healing of wounds
- Skin issues
- Loss of appetite and weight loss
- Diarrhoea
- Lethargy

Copper

Copper is the third-most abundant mineral in the body and is present in every tissue. It is stored primarily in the liver, with smaller amounts found in the brain, heart, kidneys and muscles. It is essential for:[13]

- Maintaining the strength of the skin, blood vessels, and connective tissues throughout the body
- Production of important proteins in the body such as haemoglobin, myelin, and melanin
- Keeping the thyroid gland functioning normally

Copper can be an antioxidant and a pro-oxidant, meaning that it can become toxic in higher than normal concentrations. It can also be neurotoxic and contribute to irritability, fear, nervousness, and learning and behavioural disorders.[15][16]

Dietary sources of copper include:[13]

- Beef, liver and other organ meats
- Oysters and other seafood
- Nuts and seeds
- Cocoa and chocolate
- Avocados
- Dark leafy green vegetables
- Cereals and legumes

If you compare the sources of zinc and copper, you can probably see how our modern diets can predispose us to copper overload and inadequate zinc intake. Vegetarians especially, are at an increased risk because plant foods tend to be much higher in copper than zinc.

Excretion of copper from the body is a relatively slow process (10% in 72 hours), which means that it can become problematic when there is an excess of it in the diet.[13] This is compounded when dietary zinc is low.

Some ways elevated copper can be detrimental to our wellbeing include:[14][15][17]

- Increased oxidative stress (which can cause damage to cells and their contents)
- Disrupted functioning of critical neurotransmitters
- Interfering with adrenal hormone production
- Disturbed zinc balance

Zinc, Copper, and Autism Severity

Numerous researchers have found correlations between low zinc and elevated copper, and ASD severity.[15][17-19]

Because an imbalance between these elements can contribute to dysregulated neurotransmitter system functioning, this can have wide-ranging behavioural and cognitive manifestations.

Thankfully, correcting the zinc-to-copper ratio is not overly complex and often has significant benefits for autistic children.[20-22] We will discuss testing your child's zinc and copper status in Chapter Six, and zinc supplementation in Chapter Eleven.

Vitamin D

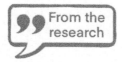

From the research

"However, there are some indications that early exposure to inadequate vitamin D may interact with other factors and contribute to the aetiology of autism, low vitamin D status might be highly prevalent in populations with ASD, and intervention with vitamin D might be beneficial in reducing autism symptoms among those who have ASD."[23]

A growing body of research is finding that autistic individuals have low levels of Vitamin D. Studies have been done with participants from Europe,[24][25] China,[26][27] the Middle East,[28-32] and the US,[33] so it seems that the problem is prevalent across the world, and not just in northern countries.

Evidence is also accumulating that there may be a link between low vitamin D status during pregnancy, foetal life, early childhood, and autism.[23]

Factors that affect your child's vitamin D status include:

- Skin pigmentation
- Where you live in the world
- Time spent in the sun and clothing worn during exposure
- Mom's vitamin D levels during pregnancy
- Intake from food and supplements

Researchers are increasingly finding links between low vitamin D status and low glutathione, and increased inflammatory and oxidative stress markers.[34][35] In other words, low vitamin D status could predispose your child to lowered antioxidant defences, and higher inflammation and oxidative damage in the body.

We know that vitamin D deficiency is also a risk factor for chronic metabolic conditions such as diabetes and cardiovascular disease, so you certainly want to improve your child's vitamin D status if it's low.

Low Omega-3 Fatty Acids

Several studies have found that children with autism have lower levels of omega-3 fatty acids than the general population.[36-40] Omega-3 fatty acids are vital for brain development and help to reduce inflammation, which is why they are one of the core five supplements to be included in your child's program. We'll revisit this topic in Chapter Ten.

Iron Deficiency

Anaemia, a common blood disorder, is an impaired ability of the blood to carry oxygen, or a decrease in the red blood cells or haemoglobin in the blood. There are many potential causes of anaemia, but the most common one is iron deficiency.

Two studies with autistic children in the US and Canada found that 8% and 16% of the participants had anaemia.[41][42] It's more common in kids under five years of age.

Iron inadequacy or deficiency can cause a variety of symptoms and issues, such as:

- Fatigue, low energy
- Shortness of breath
- Headache
- Pale skin
- Growth and development problems
- Increases absorption of the toxic metals cadmium, lead, and aluminium[5][6][43]

Another way iron deficiency can manifest itself is excessive restlessness, frequent limb jerks, and restless legs during sleep.[44] If you notice these in your child, it could serve as a clue to get their iron tested. In any case, testing iron and ferritin (the protein which stores iron in the body) should be part of the basic tests your clinician runs.

Mitochondrial Dysfunction

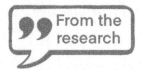

"Individuals with ASD who also have mitochondrial dysfunction are reported to have more severe behavioral and cognitive disabilities and are prone to neurodevelopmental regression compared to those with ASD without mitochondrial dysfunction."[45]

To recap what we discussed in Chapter One, mitochondria are the tiny organelles in our cells whose primary function is to produce energy (though they have other important jobs). They do this by burning (oxidising) glucose and fatty acids to produce ATP (adenosine triphosphate), which is the molecule we use to "carry" energy in the body.

Cells that have higher energy demands, such as those in the brain, gastrointestinal tract, and muscles, have more mitochondria than cells that do not have such high energy needs (e.g. skin cells).

Apart from energy production, mitochondria are involved in many other vital functions, including the life cycle of cells, steroid hormone synthesis, calcium metabolism, and neurotransmitter release.[46]

Research is increasingly showing that a large subset of autistic individuals have abnormalities in mitochondrial function, making it one of the most prevalent metabolic disturbances in ASD.[45-52]

Let's take a deeper look into the subject.

What is Mitochondrial Dysfunction?

Mitochondrial dysfunction can be classified as either primary or secondary. The basic differences are:[47]

- **Primary mitochondrial dysfunction** generally refers to mitochondrial dysfunction caused by a defect in a gene directly involved in the function of mitochondrial systems responsible for producing energy (ATP). This is often classified as mitochondrial *disease* in the medical world.
- **Secondary mitochondrial dysfunction** refers to other metabolic or genetic abnormalities (outside the mitochondria) that impair the ability of mitochondria to produce energy. We'll look at what can cause this type of secondary dysfunction in just a minute.

Effects of Mitochondrial Dysfunction in the Body

Since our mitochondria are responsible for making most of the energy we use throughout the day, if they are dysfunctional in any way, it can have serious effects on our cells' abilities to do their jobs.

Furthermore, because they are more numerous in cells that have high energy needs, such as in the brain, gut, or muscles, those cells are likely to be affected first when we have dysfunction in our mitochondria.

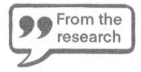

"Thus, in individuals with disorders of mitochondrial function, their most affected body organs and systems are those that have the highest energy demand, including the central and peripheral nervous system, GI tract, muscles, and immune system. Interestingly, these are some of the same organs and systems commonly affected in children with ASD."[46]

Mitochondrial disorders have recently been implicated in many neurological, neurodegenerative, and psychiatric conditions, so it's no surprise they also play a role in ASD. Some researchers have found biomarkers of mitochondrial dysfunction (such as low carnitine and elevated lactate) to correlate with more severe ASD.[53]

Other consequences of mitochondrial dysfunction can include:[46][47]

- Impairments in the detoxification systems
- Impairment of the gut and blood-brain barriers
- Increases in oxidative stress (which can further impair mitochondrial function, causing a vicious cycle)
- Diminished or disturbed neurotransmitter release
- Disturbed cellular function (fatty acid metabolism, signalling, and repair processes)
- May contribute to seizure disorders

Again, if our cells don't have energy to do their duties, all sorts of problems can arise in the body. The compounding effects of this can be significant. As one paper put it:

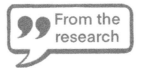

"... adding mitochondrial dysfunction to a metabolic system that is already under high oxidative stress can result in the initiation of a vicious cycle that progressively impairs cellular function, leading to neurodegeneration, regression or failure of cognitive systems to properly develop."[47]

What Factors Contribute to Mitochondrial Dysfunction?

Our mitochondria are highly sensitive to external and internal toxins and stressors, such as heavy metals, chemicals, medications, immune activation, and other metabolic disturbances.[45]

Mitochondria cannot make the antioxidant glutathione by themselves, so are dependent on the glutathione manufactured in the cell. If glutathione in the cell is depleted for any reason (e.g. oxidative stress, toxin exposure), it can negatively impact the mitochondria.

The following factors can impair mitochondrial function or increase their vulnerability to damage:[45][47]

- Malnutrition (e.g. vitamin B_6, folate, coenzyme Q_{10}, iron, or haem deficiencies)
- Glutathione depletion or deficiency
- Oxidative stress
- Heavy metals and chemicals (e.g. pesticides, PCBs)
- Bacterial, yeast, or mould toxins (e.g. LPS, mycotoxins)
- Some medications (e.g. antibiotics, proton-pump inhibitors, valproic acid, acetaminophen)
- Certain short-chain fatty acids, such as propionate (discussed in Chapter Three)
- Imbalances in the excitatory and inhibitory neurotransmitter systems (see the section Excess Glutamate and Excitotoxicity in this chapter)
- Inflammation caused by immune activation

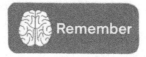

Remember, due to many of the above-listed factors, your child's mitochondria may be more vulnerable to environmental toxins than if they were otherwise healthy. A combination of these stressors may have even more adverse effects. This is why the second part of this book will go into great detail on how you can address as many of them as possible.

What Can Be Done?

When mitochondrial disorders are caused by environmental factors rather than genetics, usually much can be done to improve the situation. Most importantly, you would need to:

- Identify and remove contributing factors (e.g. toxic burden)
- Identify and address contributing metabolic abnormalities (e.g. carnitine deficiency)
- Support your child's mitochondria with antioxidants and nutritional co-factors.

We'll revisit this topic in Chapter Six, Eleven and Twelve, where we'll discuss:

- Physical clues that may indicate your child has mitochondrial dysfunction
- Markers on the organic acids test that may indicate mitochondrial dysfunction
- Blood test markers your doctor can use to investigate further
- Supplements that can support the mitochondria

Carnitine Deficiency

Carnitine is a compound that carries long-chain fatty acids into the mitochondria, where they can be "burned-up" to produce energy. It also carries potentially toxic substances out of the mitochondria so the cells can excrete them. Because it is so important for energy production, depleted carnitine levels can contribute to mitochondrial dysfunction. As it happens, numerous studies have reported sub-optimal or deficient carnitine levels in autistic children over the years.[47][53-55]

We'll talk about carnitine supplementation in Chapter Eleven.

Glutathione Status

As the primary antioxidant in the body, glutathione has many critical jobs to do, including:

- Binding toxic metals and chemicals (so they can be excreted in bile or urine)
- Supporting the immune and nervous systems, gastrointestinal tract, and the lungs
- Helping to recycle other antioxidants such as vitamin C and E
- Supporting DNA synthesis and repair
- Indirectly supporting protein synthesis

When glutathione is depleted, because of increased toxic burden or impaired production, a lot of damage can happen in the body due to oxidative stress. Many researchers have shown glutathione to be low in autistic children.[56-69]

We will discuss strategies to reduce factors that deplete glutathione and nutrients to support its production in Part Two of the book.

Impaired Methylation

Impaired methylation can lead to problems with the immune and hormonal systems, detoxification, energy production, and countless other vital processes in the body.

We don't need to get too technical - this book is not intended to do that. Just think of it as a cycle that needs to keep running. Various nutrients and steps are required to keep the cycle going smoothly. If a nutrient is missing or there is a blockage somewhere in the cycle, it can back up the previous steps. This can cause a build-up of certain compounds that can be harmful in excess or can hinder important processes in the body. It also means that steps later in the cycle don't get their needed materials, so they can't do their jobs properly.

Many researchers have found methylation to be impaired in autistic children.[58-60][63][68][70] What can disrupt your child's methylation capacities? Some common causes include:

- Genetic variations (e.g. MTHFR gene polymorphisms)
- Certain nutrient deficiencies or imbalances (e.g. vitamin B_{12} and folate deficiencies)
- Oxidative stress and inflammation
- Heavy metals and chemical toxins
- Pathogens

Are you starting to see a pattern emerging here? The same culprits keep coming up again and again. This is why Part Two of the *Autism Wellbeing Plan* focuses on addressing them. You can refer to Chapter Eleven for a list of supplements that can be used to support methylation.

Excess Glutamate and Excitotoxicity

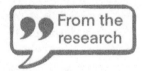

"Increased glutamate may be linked to some of the behavioral problems and features commonly associated with autism."[4]

Glutamate is the most abundant neurotransmitter in the central nervous system. It plays important roles in brain development, learning, memory, gene expression, taste, and skin pain sensation (to name a few).[4][71][72]

In excess, however, glutamate has been shown to be a potent neurotoxin.[72] Many studies have reported elevated glutamate levels in autistic individuals, and some researchers consider disrupted glutamate metabolism to play an important role in the development of ASD.[71-74]

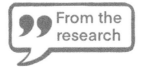

"Moreover, we suggest that the increasing prevalence of ASD during the last decades might reflect the synergistic action of increased burden of new ecotoxicological factors, which include excitotoxic amino acids, mainly glutamate and aspartate, fluoride in combination with aluminum (Al3+), mercury, and the increasing number of vaccines in the period of rapid postnatal brain development."[71]

Elevated glutamate levels have also been reported in other conditions, including major depressive disorder, obsessive-compulsive disorder (OCD), social anxiety disorder, and epilepsy.[73] Coincidently, these are common comorbid conditions with ASD.

Glutamate can get converted to GABA (gamma-aminobutyric acid), which is a calming (inhibitory) neurotransmitter. Studies have reported that there is often a failure to make this conversion in autistic children, and this imbalance can lead to stimming behaviours (due to too much neuronal excitation) and speech impairment in some kids (due to too little GABA).[15][73]

Other potential problems excess glutamate can cause include:[71][75]

- Glutathione depletion (and its many knock-on effects)
- Can be a causative factor in seizures
- Disruption of the blood-brain barrier
- Inhibiting the release of the sleep-regulating hormone melatonin from the pineal gland

What is Excitotoxicity?

Too much glutamate in the brain and central nervous system can lead to what is known as excitotoxicity. This is a process that can cause damage to, or even kill, brain cells and nervous system tissue. Excitotoxicity causes oxidative stress, mitochondrial damage, and can play a role in neurodegeneration.[4]

It is common in many disorders, including epilepsy, strokes, brain trauma, autoimmunity, heavy metal toxicity, and the majority of neurodegenerative diseases.[75]

Factors that can disrupt glutamate balance or trigger excitotoxicity include:[46][71]

- Excessive immune activation (which can cause chronic brain inflammation)
- Mitochondrial dysfunction
- Elevated copper, low zinc
- Activation of microglia (discussed in Chapter Two)
- Dietary excitotoxins (e.g. MSG, aspartame)
- Mercury, aluminium, and fluoride
- Magnesium deficiency
- Genetic variations

As you can see, food and the metals or additives that often contaminate it can greatly contribute to excitotoxicity. We'll take a closer look at MSG, mercury, aluminium, fluoride, and how they can undermine your child's health in the next chapter.

In Part Two, I'll discuss strategies to reduce dietary excitotoxins and supplements that can help mitigate the effects of this harmful process.

Sulphate and Sulphation Impairments

Sulphur (sulfur in American English) is the fourth most common mineral in the human body. It's used for many functions including detoxification, maintaining the gut lining, synthesis of brain tissue, and neurotransmitter metabolism.

The process of sulphation (sulfation, if you're in the US) is too complex to get into here, but suffice it to say that, like methylation, it's absolutely critical that it runs well in the body. Otherwise, imbalances start happening.

For example, impairments in sulphation can lead to diminished detoxification, which allows heavy metals such as mercury to build up in the body.[76]

Various reasons exist for impairments in sulphation:

- Poor absorption of sulphate in the gut
- Excess loss of sulphate in the urine
- Poor recycling of sulphate in the kidneys

- Nutrient deficiencies (e.g. molybdenum)
- Oxidative stress
- Inflammation
- Presence of sulphate-reducing bacteria (e.g. *Desulfovibrio*)
- Chemical toxicity (e.g. glyphosate)

We'll discuss a couple of strategies you can use to replenish your child's sulphate in Chapter Eleven.

Elevated Oxalate Levels

Oxalate, or oxalic acid, is a highly acidic organic acid that can bind with minerals such as calcium and magnesium to form crystals. It has been found to be high in autistic children[83] and is often elevated when they are tested with the organic acids test.

Oxalates are found in many foods, are produced by certain fungi, and are sometimes formed naturally in our bodies. Ordinarily, we only absorb a fraction of dietary oxalates, but when the gut is inflamed and leaky, as is often the case in ASD, oxalate absorption can increase dramatically.

Oxalate crystals can form in the bones, joints, kidneys, blood vessels, lungs, thyroid, and even the brain, which can impede their proper function or cause pain. In fact, calcium oxalate is the major component of the most common kidney stones. Autistic children that exhibit eye poking behaviours should certainly be tested for elevated oxalate levels.

An increased oxalate burden in the body can:

- Deplete glutathione
- Increase oxidative stress
- Inhibit absorption of essential minerals such as calcium, magnesium, zinc, and iron
- Bind with heavy metals and trap them in the body

The best way to test your child for elevated oxalates is using the organic acids test from the Great Plains Laboratory (see Chapter Six). I discuss what to do about high oxalates in Chapter Seven, Eleven, and Twelve.

What Can You Do About It?

In Part Two of the *Autism Wellbeing Plan*, we will discuss strategies to:

- Test your child's nutrient status
- Spot clues that mitochondrial dysfunction may be present
- Test for oxalates and what to do if they are elevated
- Balance zinc and copper
- Support mitochondrial function
- Support glutathione production
- Support methylation
- Replenish sulphate
- Reduce excitotoxicity
- And much more

Wrap-up

We covered a lot of ground in this chapter. I started by explaining why most autistic children need a comprehensive and well-designed supplementation program to support them on their journey to improved wellbeing. We looked at how certain nutrient deficiencies can increase your child's susceptibility to toxic metals. You saw that research around the world has shown autistic kids' diets to be low in various essential nutrients.

Much of our focus in this chapter was to give you an overview of the many nutritional and metabolic imbalances that often afflict autistic children, and some consequences they can have. We concluded the chapter with a reminder that we'll consider strategies to address the imbalances we discussed in Part Two of the *Autism Wellbeing Plan*.

In the next chapter, we turn to the topic of environmental toxins and the role they can play in diminishing your child's health.

CHAPTER FIVE: HEAVY METALS AND CHEM-ICAL TOXICITY

Overview of This Chapter

We're nearly there. This is the last chapter in Part One, but its importance cannot be overstated, as you will soon see.

The main points I will cover are:

- Why kids are more vulnerable to toxins than adults
- The myriad of ways in which toxic substances can harm us
- A brief look at research linking heavy metals and ASD severity
- The five most prevalent heavy metals in our environment, their sources of exposure, and some ways they can do damage to the body
- The most common man-made chemicals, food additives, and pollutants you'll need to learn how to avoid (the practical aspects of which will be discussed in Chapter Eight)

Kids Are More Vulnerable to Toxic Insults

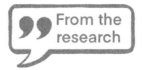

"In a colossal toxicological experiment carried out over the last few decades, there has been the unprecedented production and release of tens of thousands of chemical agents into the environment without sufficient consideration for human safety and without credible testing to secure the absence of danger or harm."[1]

It should come as no surprise to you that we live in the most polluted time of our human existence - and it's taking its toll on us all. From pesticide residues on our food, and chemicals in everyday products, to the car exhausts we breathe in daily - no one can truly escape the toxic onslaught with which we are faced. The best we can do is learn how to mitigate it. But babies and young children are the most vulnerable for these reasons:

- Their detoxification capacities are still not fully developed
- The protective blood-brain barrier is not fully formed until about six months of age
- Their behaviours (e.g. crawling on the ground, mouthing objects) puts them at higher risk of ingesting harmful substances
- Relatively speaking, children consume more food and water per unit of body weight than adults, which amplifies their daily toxic burden (lower exposures can have a stronger effect than would on an adult)

So, children in general are more vulnerable, can absorb toxins more rapidly, and those toxins are cleared more slowly than in adults. As if that's not challenging enough to deal with, in the case of autistic children, further problems can rear their ugly head, such as:

- Impaired detoxification capacities

- Increased oxidative stress
- Increased leaky gut
- Disrupted gut microbiota
- Depleted glutathione and other antioxidants
- In some cases, increased exposure to toxins
- Genetic factors may also predispose some children to increased vulnerability to toxic compounds

Some or all of the above factors can conspire to sabotage your child's health. It's key to note that strong, acute exposure is not necessary to have a negative effect on your child. Even small exposures over time can be devastating, for the reasons I mentioned above.

How Toxins Harm Us

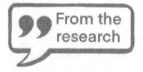

"In addition, chain reactions of metabolic disruption might occur as one toxic action may prompt another and then another, resulting in a cascade of altered outcomes. For example, toxic chemical agents may induce oxidative stress which may result in mitochondrial damage, which may prevent normal cell demise, which may produce inflammatory changes in tissues, which may cause maldigestion or malabsorption in the gastrointestinal tract and subsequent nutritional compromise with assorted signs and symptoms."[1]

I think you will agree that the myriad of ways toxins can do damage to the body is truly staggering. Below are some of the main mechanisms through which heavy metals and toxic chemicals can harm us:[1]

- Damage cells and their components or organelles (e.g. cell membranes, nucleus, DNA, mitochondria)

- Interfere with energy production
- Affect gene expression and DNA repair
- Interfere with critical enzymes
- Contribute to oxidative stress
- Disturb the hormone systems of the body
- Disrupt the gut microbiota
- Cause neurotransmitter disturbances
- Interfere with methylation
- Disturb communication between cells or organs
- Cause immune reactions, inflammation, and antibody formation
- Contribute to immune dysfunction, dysregulation, and autoimmunity
- Impair detoxification pathways
- Displace nutrients in enzymes or receptor sites
- Dysregulate the nervous system

Many toxins bio-accumulate in our tissues. They can get sequestered in fat cells, but they can also end up in our organs, including the brain.

Some chemicals, such as BPA and phthalates, are what we call endocrine disrupting chemicals (EDCs). Endocrine refers to the body's hormonal systems, which means that EDCs disrupt the function of the body's hormones. This is, of course, a bad thing because they can affect the thyroid gland, adrenal function, sexual maturation, and countless other critical metabolic processes.[1]

Many compounds are neurotoxic - they damage brain and nervous system tissues. Examples include mercury, lead, solvents, pesticides, and EDCs.[2]

The worst part is that toxins can exert serious damage at seemingly minuscule doses. Just because you can't see them, doesn't mean they aren't affecting your family. As adults, we often won't feel the effects of significant toxic exposures. But autistic kids are much more sensitive to their environment than most people can imagine. That is, in part, why their symptoms can fluctuate so much from day to day.

We know very little on how multiple toxins work synergistically to wreak havoc in the body because scant research has been done in this area. Who would fund it? The producers of these chemicals? They have no incentive to do so. It's unfathomably careless and extremely dangerous to just release them into our world, but that's precisely what the regulatory agencies are allowing to happen.

Research is emerging that indicates that toxin exposure could be contributing to the increase in autism, both in influencing its development and its severity. For example, one recent study found strong associations between body burden of various organic pollutants and ASD severity.[3]

As further investigation is done in this area, my hope is that we can spread awareness to more families of the dangers hidden in many innocent-looking products we use on a daily basis. I'm talking about everything from our food and water, to the soaps, cleaning products, and plastics that are all part of modern life.

Overview of Our Toxic Landscape

We'll focus the rest of this chapter on giving you an overview of the most prevalent toxins in our environment. You don't need to be an expert on the subject to help your child, but I want you to have a better understanding of what you're up against. That way, when I recommend certain lifestyle or dietary changes later, you won't think I'm some over-zealous toxin-phobe. As you will soon see, our modern lifestyle and environment are a minefield you need to learn to navigate.

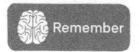

As you read on, please try not to get disheartened. It may seem overwhelming, but remember that we'll discuss practical strategies to clean up your child's diet and environment in Part Two of the book. In many cases, simple broad-sweeping actions on your part can have tremendous impact on reducing your entire family's toxic burden. The best example is switching to an all-organic diet. By doing that alone, you reduce an unthinkable amount of exposure to herbicides, pesticides, artificial fertilisers, hormones, genetically modified crops, and who-knows-what-else they put in our food nowadays.

For the purposes of our discussion, we'll divide toxins into two broad categories: heavy metals and man-made chemicals.

Heavy Metals in More Depth

Heavy metals are naturally occurring components in the Earth's crust. On the one hand, this is a good thing (when comparing them to man-made chemicals) because our bodies have been exposed to them since the dawn of humanity - thus, we've adapted to detoxify and excrete them.

The problem nowadays, in our heavily industrialised society, is that human activities are causing an inordinate amount of heavy metals to be released into the environment. These metals end up in the air, water, soil, food supply, and in our bodies.

In fact, *every* single person whose hair I've had tested, from the age of 2 to 58, has *at the very least* had significant amounts of mercury and aluminium coming out of them. I would be more worried if I didn't see some heavy metals on a hair test - it can often mean the person's detoxification systems are not working as well as they should.

The danger with heavy metals is that if we don't have the capacity to excrete them as fast as they come in, they will bio-accumulate in our vital organs and other tissues. Kids with impaired detoxification ability due to genetics, oxidative stress, or other factors will be at much higher risk of toxicity.

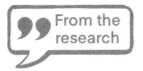

From the research

"Interestingly, the severity of autism could be well correlated with the level of accumulation of toxic elements like Pb [lead] and Hg [mercury]. LFA [low-functioning autism] showed significantly higher accumulation of toxic elements like Pb and Hg in the hair and nail when compared with HFA [high-functioning autism]. LFA also showed a significant decrease in the concentration of trace metals like Mg [magnesium] and Se [selenium] in the hair and nail when compared to HFA."[4] (Note: comments in square brackets added by the author.)

Research on Heavy Metals and Autism Severity

Many researchers have found elevations of toxic metals in the hair, urine, and blood of autistic children. The most common metals detected are mercury, lead, aluminium, arsenic, and cadmium. Others such as antimony, nickel, vanadium, uranium, tin, thallium, and tungsten have also been detected.[5-7]

Relatively few studies have looked at heavy metal levels and tried to correlate them to autism severity. The few that have, however, seem to find at least some connection between heavy metal status and ASD severity. Overall, there is compelling evidence that toxic metals influence autism severity, at least in a subset of children.[4][8] We'll briefly review some notable studies here.

One group of researchers found that higher body burden of heavy metals was associated with more severe autistic symptoms in two studies.[7][9] In one of the studies, they found that lead, antimony, mercury, tin, and aluminium were most associated with autism severity.[9] In the second paper, the authors stated:[7]

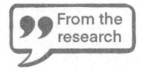
From the research

"However, in autism, the problem appears to usually not be high exposure, but rather decreased excretion. The half-life of lead, mercury, and other toxic metals in the blood is weeks to months, so those metals rapidly leave the blood and accumulate in tissue and/or bone."[7]

Other researchers found more severe autism to be correlated with elevated mercury and copper. They also found that lead was associated with a decrease in IQ in their study.[10]

Another study found high aluminium, arsenic, cadmium, mercury, antimony, nickel, lead, and vanadium in autistic children. Most notably, mercury, lead, and nickel correlated with ASD symptom severity.[6]

Finally, a paper reported that metabolites associated with mercury or lead toxicity (called porphyrins) detected in the urine of autistic children were significantly associated with CARS scores. In other words, study participants with more severe ASD scores tended to have higher levels of those compounds in their urine.[11] The researchers also found lower levels of compounds needed to detoxify heavy metals in the ASD group (glutathione, cysteine, and sulphate). Can you see how increased heavy metal burden, low glutathione, and impaired sulphation could affect an autistic child?

The "Big Five" Heavy Metals

There are about two dozen heavy metals to which we have meaningful exposure in our daily lives. In this section we'll take a closer look at the five most prevalent ones, namely:

- Mercury
- Aluminium
- Arsenic
- Lead
- Cadmium

The Agency for Toxic Substances and Disease Registry (ATSDR) in the United States ranks four of these metals in the top 10 of their Substance Priority List, with arsenic, lead, and mercury taking first, second and third position respectively in the list in 2017 (and cadmium being in seventh position).[12]

Needless to say, these metals are a serious risk to public health all around the world, and knowing what we're up against is the first step in reducing the damage they do to our families.

Mercury

Exposure to mercury begins in the womb and continues throughout our lives. No one can really avoid it. All we can hope for is to minimise the damage it can do by avoiding it as much as possible and supporting our natural detoxification systems.

Common sources of exposure include:

- In the air
- Large fish
- Cleaning products
- Pharmaceuticals
- Fertilisers

- Fungicides
- Coal burning for energy production

There are various forms of mercury, both organic and inorganic, which carry different concerns. One organic form of it, ethyl mercury (thimerosal is an infamous example) is used in fish farming and many medications due to its strong anti-bacterial and anti-fungal properties.[13]

Organic mercury has the dangerous ability to cross the blood-brain barrier, where it can bind to tissues and damage the brain and central nervous system. Toxicity can cause all kinds of problems, from neurological issues and cardiovascular or respiratory complications, to impaired kidney function and immune system abnormalities.[5][14]

In fact, mercury poisoning and autism have nearly identical symptoms, such as:[15]

- Self-injurious behaviour
- Social withdrawal
- Lack of eye contact
- Lack of facial expression
- Hypersensitivity to noise and touch
- Repetitive behaviours

Of course, that's talking about acute toxicity. The effects of chronic, low-level toxicity are much more insidious. Many autistic children have trouble detoxifying mercury due to reasons we've already discussed, which can make even "typical for our world" exposures have a meaningful effect on their health.

Mercury can:[1][16-18]

- Deplete glutathione
- Trigger excitotoxicity
- Interfere with glutamate metabolism
- Inhibit important enzymes in the body
- Contribute to oxidative stress
- Damage the blood-brain barrier
- Damage cell membranes
- Disrupt the methylation process in cells
- Contribute to autoimmunity

Aluminium

Many studies have demonstrated the toxic effect of aluminium (aluminum in the US) on the gut, musculoskeletal, and nervous systems, with the end result often being autoimmunity or neuroautoimmunity.[19]

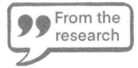

"Despite this knowledge, aluminum continues to be used in food products, food packaging and vaccines, where it may contribute to the autoimmune epidemic we currently face."[19]

Aluminium is the third most common naturally occurring element on Earth (after oxygen and silicone) and is therefore ubiquitous in the air, water, soil, and food supply. Unfortunately, it is also intentionally added to many foods (including baby formula and cosmetic products).[16]

Common sources of exposure:

- In the air, water, and food
- Used as an anti-caking agent (in flour, table salt, baking soda)
- Used in some food additives, such as emulsifiers
- Aluminium cookware
- Food and beverage cans
- Some snacks, desserts, and baked goods
- Exhaust fumes
- Cosmetics (e.g. antiperspirants)
- Vaccines

Like mercury, aluminium can also bind to human tissues and instigate a chain reaction of immune responses which can lead to autoimmunity.[16] It can accumulate in the brain and produce inflammation by various mechanisms, including microglial activation, oxidative stress, and the damaging of cell membranes.[17][20]

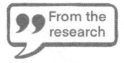

"Based on vaccine product insert information and the CDC recommended vaccination schedule, at 12 and 18 months of age, babies receive around 1500 and 6000 micrograms of aluminum respectively. Being that the human body, immune system, vital organs and tissues are still developing during this fragile age, does it make sense to knowingly inject aluminum into our children?"[19]

I'm glad at least some researchers are questioning why we allow tiny, fragile human beings to be injected with aluminium. It's one thing to get it in our food or water - at least we have various mechanisms to protect us. Depending on how leaky our gut is, only a fraction may make it into the body. But when you inject it directly into the blood, the aluminium is many steps closer to finding its way to the brain and nervous system. Clearly, we should be investigating safer adjuvants to use in vaccines. Let's hope the research catches up with current practices.

Arsenic

One in-depth analysis of arsenic, cadmium, and manganese exposure in neurodevelopmental and behavioural disorders in children found:

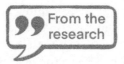

"In 13 of the 15 articles studied, we found that arsenic exposure had a significant negative effect on neurodevelopment in children aged between 5 and 15 years. In most studies, this deleterious effect affected Full Scale IQ. More specifically, a deficit was found in verbal and per formance domains, with memory being affected to a lesser extent"[21]

To put it more simply, arsenic was found to have a negative effect on children's IQ in most of the studies that were reviewed.

Arsenic exposure has harmful effects on many of the body's organs and systems, including the gut, liver, kidneys, skin, blood, and nervous and immune systems.[21] It's a whole-system poison, and probably the reason why it was such a popular means to assassinate people in our past history. Nowadays it can be detected in hair, so it has lost its attractiveness for such purposes.

Arsenic can cause damage to the brain and central nervous system, which explains why it is associated with impaired neurodevelopment and behavioural disorders in children. Its neurotoxic effects can contribute to:[22]

- Learning disability
- Memory impairment
- Disorders of the brain (encephalopathy)
- Psychomotor problems (e.g. problems with movement, coordination, fine and gross motor skills)

Other significant ways arsenic can interfere with health include:[5]

- Contributing to oxidative stress
- Disturbing DNA repair processes
- Interference with important enzymes in the body

Most of the adverse effects of arsenic are thought to be caused by its interference with enzymes used for energy production in our cells.[22] This makes sense because if the cells themselves can't produce enough energy, then they can't do their jobs, which may include getting rid of toxins, supplying nutrients to organs, repairing DNA or other important structures, or otherwise keeping us alive and healthy.

Because arsenic is so abundant in the Earth's crust, some exposure is inevitable, as plants absorb many metals from the soil as they grow. Human activities that contribute to the release of arsenic into the environment include burning of fossil fuels, mining, smelting, waste incineration, and use of herbicides and pesticides.[21][22]

The drinking water of many countries is contaminated, making it the biggest source of arsenic exposure for millions of children across the world. Some high-risk countries include Argentina, Chile, Mexico, China, Hungary, India, Bangladesh, and Vietnam.[21]

Common sources of exposure:

- In the air and water
- Non-organic chicken and eggs
- Non-organic rice and rice products
- Can be found in fish, fruits and vegetables
- Pesticides and fungicides
- Cosmetics
- Wood preservatives

Lead

Governments around the world have been working to remove lead from petrol, paint, and soldered cans, but exposure is still a major public health problem. Lead is one of the most abundant metals in the Earth's crust, so traces of it will invariably be found in the soil, air, and some water sources. Certain geographic regions have higher levels in the soil and environment due to past use of lead as a petrol and paint additive.

Lead poisoning in children can cause serious problems with growth and mental development.[5] Younger kids are especially susceptible to exposure because of their crawling and mouthing behaviours. High lead levels have been associated with:[23]

- Negative effects on development and cognitive ability
- Learning and behavioural disabilities
- ADHD (attention deficit hyperactivity disorder)
- Behavioural disturbances

This is not surprising, given that lead interferes with the metabolism of neurotransmitters such as dopamine and GABA, which can have wide-ranging behavioural effects.[24]

Common sources of lead exposure include:

- In the air
- Contaminated water
- May be present in some soils
- Some paints, varnishes, and similar products
- Coal burning for energy and other
- Industrial emissions

You know by now that relatively low exposure to a toxin, especially when coupled with reduced ability to detoxify it, can still cause significant negative effects on your child's health. You may also remember from the previous chapter that calcium, iron, and zinc deficiencies can increase lead absorption.[24][25]

Cadmium

Cadmium toxicity has been associated with neurological and behavioural disorders. It has also been shown to cause damage or dysfunction in the brain, liver, kidneys, lungs, testis, bones, and even the placenta.[5][26]

Some ways cadmium may harm our health include:[5][24-27]

- Disturbs the blood-brain barrier
- Contributing to oxidative stress in the brain
- Inducing apoptosis, which triggers the death of cells
- Causes neurotransmitter disturbances
- Disturbs the metabolism of essential minerals such as calcium, zinc, and iron

Cadmium is used in many industrial and household products, such as batteries, metal coatings, plastics, ceramics and glass, some metal alloys, and pigments.[21][26] Apart from industry (but largely due to industry contaminating our environment), cadmium is found in nearly all foods to a degree, though plant foods tend to be higher in it.[27]

Common sources of exposure include:

- Contaminated soil or water
- Large ocean fish
- Seafood such as shellfish, oysters, crab, and octopus
- Fertilisers, fungicides
- Air pollution, exhaust fumes
- Processed and refined foods (e.g. processed meats, cola drinks)
- Coal burning
- Cigarette smoke (including indirect exposure)

Exposure to cadmium tends to be higher in Asian countries (such as China and Japan) than in Europe and the USA, due to the rapid growth of industries causing cadmium pollution and the high intake of rice grown on contaminated soil.[27]

Man-Made Chemicals and Additives

There are literally tens of thousands of chemicals that have been manufactured in the last century. Of those, an infinitesimally tiny portion have been studied for their toxic effects on humans. Additionally, it takes an *inordinate* amount of proof to convince regulatory agencies to ban harmful substances.

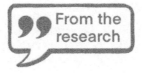

From the research

"The two main impediments to prevention of neurodevelopmental deficits of chemical origin are the great gaps in testing chemicals for developmental neurotoxicity and the high level of proof required for regulation. New, precautionary approaches that recognise the unique vulnerability of the developing brain are needed for testing and control of chemicals."[2]

In this section, I'll cover some of the most prevalent chemicals and additives that can harm your child. The list is so vast that we will barely scratch the surface. Some of the most common exposures are to:

- Herbicides and pesticides
- Plastics and plasticisers (e.g. BPA and phthalates)
- Food additives (e.g. artificial colours, flavours, emulsifiers, preservatives)
- Fluoride and chlorine additives in water
- Fire retardants
- Chemicals in household cleaning products
- Chemicals in sunscreen
- Air pollution is a major source of toxic exposure

Let's take a closer look at some of the above.

Herbicides and Pesticides

Herbicides, pesticides, and fungicides are designed to kill living organisms by poisoning them in some way. That alone should be a major red flag. As you'll see, these chemicals contaminate our environment on a colossal scale and have the most insidious pathway to harm us - our food.

Glyphosate - The Most Prevalent Herbicide

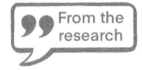

"Glyphosate works synergistically with other factors, such as insufficient sun exposure, dietary deficiencies in critical nutrients such as sulfur and zinc, and synergistic exposure to other xenobiotics whose detoxification is impaired by glyphosate."[16]

You may have heard of the infamous herbicide RoundUp®. Glyphosate is the active ingredient in it, and now that the patent has expired, manufacturers around the world are producing enormous quantities of it every year. This means that farmers are spraying millions of tons of it on their crops.

Though glyphosate has been around since the 1960s, its use increased dramatically in the 90s, as glyphosate-tolerant genetically modified (GM) crops were heavily marketed to farmers.

The use of glyphosate does not end with GM crops. It is also used as a desiccant. Some farmers spray it on crops (including wheat and other non-GM crops) just before harvest to dry them out and prevent them from spoiling or sprouting. This further increases the prevalence of this chemical in our food supply.

In the US, glyphosate has been detected in many popular breakfast foods, including some organic products, which is worrying. (Contamination is always a risk, but this doesn't mean organic foods are not worth the investment.) Glyphosate use in Europe is lower than the US, however it has been shown to be present in cereals, bread, beer, as well as in the urine and even breast milk of humans.[28][29]

Early short-term studies showed little toxicity in rats, which gave everyone, including farmers, regulators, and homeowners, a false sense of security about the safety of this herbicide. However, longer-term studies are showing that it's not harmless - quite the opposite, in fact.[16]

One of the primary ways that glyphosate harms us is by disrupting our gut bacteria - the beneficial ones in particular. As you know by now, this causes a negative chain reaction throughout the whole body by allowing pathogens to overgrow, causing dysbiosis, leaky gut and inflammation, and the subsequent immune reactions.

More precisely, glyphosate inhibits an enzyme in plants, bacteria, and fungi that inhibits a process (the shikimate pathway) used to produce the amino acids tyrosine, tryptophan and phenylalanine.

Why is that important? For one, these amino acids are the precursors for important neurotransmitters and hormones such as dopamine, serotonin, melatonin, adrenaline, and noradrenaline. Some of these are made in our gut by our bacteria. By disturbing our microbiota, glyphosate can disturb our neurotransmitter and hormone balance. At this point in the book, I'm sure you understand that the ramifications of this can be far-reaching and harmful elsewhere in the body, including the brain.

There are other mechanisms of action through which glyphosate may harm us. These include:[16][30-33]

- Binding to human tissues to form neo-antigens that can instigate immune and autoimmune responses
- Interfering with sulphate metabolism
- Causing oxidative stress
- Binding minerals such as zinc, iron, calcium, magnesium, and manganese, making them unavailable to the body

Much research still needs to be done in this area, but we have more than enough reasons to steer clear of foods which may be sprayed with this dangerous chemical.

Still need more convincing? Glyphosate was classified as a "probable human carcinogen" (i.e. cancer-causing) in March 2015 by the International Agency for Research on Cancer (IARC), which is the specialised cancer agency of the World Health Organization (WHO).[34]

This was a step in the right direction, and since then a number of countries moved to ban glyphosate. There are now at least 19 countries that have banned or restricted its use.[35]

Germany announced in September 2019 that glyphosate will be

banned by 2023 and begun to be phased out from 2020.

I wish I had better tidings to report from the USA, though. Despite the WHO statement in 2015 and the banning of it in various countries, the Environmental Protection Agency (EPA) announced in May 2019 that it proposed to re-approve glyphosate after its own internal review.[36] An EPA administrator said: "EPA has found no risks to public health from the current registered uses of glyphosate".

Obviously, a very backward move which reeks of corruption and complete disregard for the health of the American public. Sad and infuriating, indeed.

All this means that you need to be extra careful if you live in the United States, because it looks like odds are stacked against you. Let us hope the continued activism of courageous scientists and concerned citizens brings about some badly needed change there.

Pesticides

Pesticides come in many sinister flavours. The large group of organophosphate pesticides (OPPs) are obviously toxic to insects, but exposure to humans is also harmful, even in small amounts.

One infamous OPP, chlorpyrifos, is still used in about 100 countries despite having been shown to cause neurodevelopmental delays and other issues.[37]

In the United States, chlorpyrifos use was banned in 2000 for certain crops and for use around homes, schools, and other places where children may be exposed.

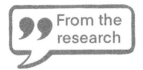
From the research

"Children exposed to higher, compared with lower, chlorpyrifos levels were also significantly more likely to experience Psychomotor Development Index and Mental Development Index delays, attention problems, attention-deficit/hyperactivity disorder problems, and pervasive developmental disorder problems at 3 years of age."[37]

In 2007, the EPA was petitioned to ban the chemical completely but after dragging its heels to make a decision, they announced in 2017 that they won't be banning it.[38][39] Another move that obviously has industry interests at heart and completely disregards public health.

This is yet another extremely important reason to buy your food organic. Do not expect your government or any other institution to protect you. Rather, take responsibility for your family's health and arm yourself with knowledge. (I'll be stressing the importance of organic food throughout Part Two.)

Some mechanisms of how pesticides may increase the risk for autism include:[40]

- Developmental neurotoxicity
- Oxidative stress
- Mitochondrial dysfunction
- Immune toxicity (e.g. immunosuppression, neuroinflammation)

Prenatal exposure is particularly dangerous because many pesticides, including OPPs, can cross the placenta.[37]

One study found that risk for ASD increased the closer pregnant women lived to sites where organochlorine pesticides were used. The risk increased with proximity to sites with pesticides and as the amount of pesticides used increased.[41]

Another study found that methyl bromide, a fungicide used in strawberry production, was associated with restricted foetal growth during pregnancy when women were in close residential proximity to it during the second trimester.[42]

Genetically Modified Foods

Genetically Modified (GM) foods are not technically chemicals, of course, but are an important piece of the puzzle, especially when talking about glyphosate (the two go hand-in-hand).

GM crops have been banned in at least 39 countries so far, 28 of which are in Europe.[43] A lot of positive progress has been made in this area, though much work remains to be done.

If you live in the United States, however, you'd better watch out because the stats are shocking. Some 90% or more of soy, canola, corn, cotton, and sugar beet crops grown there are genetically modified. Not to mention that labelling isn't required for foods that contain GM ingredients.

Did you know that GM foods are not even tested on humans before being let loose into the market?

Aside from heavy use of glyphosate and pesticides, other problems with GM foods include the fact that altering the genetics of plants can lead to unpredictable changes in their expression. This can cause new toxins and allergens to be expressed in the plant.

In some cases, the GM plant is engineered to become an insecticide itself. One example is Bt toxin crops where the plant is made to express a protein that the bacteria *Bacillus thuringiensis* produces. When a bug eats the plant's leaves, the toxin causes its gut to get punctured so the bacteria that live in the insect invade it, eventually causing it to die from the infection.

Sounds lovely, doesn't it? Please stay away from GM foods if you can help it and be especially careful with processed products. The best way to avoid genetically modified ingredients is to stick to certified organic foods.

Food Additives

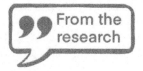

"Glucose, salt, emulsifiers, organic solvents, gluten, microbial transglutaminase, and nanoparticles are extensively and increasingly used by the food industry, claim the manufacturers, to improve the qualities of food. However, all of the aforementioned additives increase intestinal permeability by breaching the integrity of tight junction paracellular transfer."[44]

Nowadays, more than 2500 additives are added to food to keep certain properties or extend shelf life.[45]

We obviously can't cover many here, but we'll touch on some of the most prevalent and insidious ones. The main takeaway is this: avoid industrial foods and cook as many meals from scratch as possible. This is the best way to protect your child from the countless chemicals that pervade our food supply. I will be echoing this advice in the rest of the book.

Table Salt

It's not salt that's bad for you, it's the processed table salt that is the culprit implicated in many diseases. In terms of mineral content, table salt consists of only sodium, chloride, and often iodine. In addition, most people are unaware that aluminium is added to table salt to keep it free-flowing and prevent it from caking.

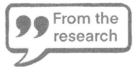

"Salt is considered a silent killer since increased consumption is associated with hypertension, strokes, left ventricular hypertrophy, renal diseases, obesity, renal stones and stomach cancer. Over consumption of salts is real, spanning multiple populations, ages, gender and continents."[44]

We're not only eating an inordinate amount of salt as a society, but that salt is in the harmful form. The largest contributor to this phenomenon is, unsurprisingly, processed food. 80% of consumed salt comes from manufactured food products in developed countries.[46]

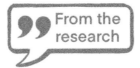

"The salt content in processed foods can be more than a 100 times higher than that in similar homemade meals."[47]

Cereals and baked goods are the largest contributor to sodium intake in UK and US adults, while soy sauce is the largest source in Asia.[44] It's likely to be similar for kids as they learn their dietary habits from their parents.

If all that isn't enough to make you stop using regular table salt, recent research has also found that salt can contribute to leaky gut and activate the immune system in potentially harmful ways.[44]

Quality sea salt is different from table salt. It has many more minerals and trace elements, thus has a much more balanced mineral profile. You can even feel it yourself that you don't feel immediately thirsty after eating some sea salt, the way you do when you eat food that contains processed table salt.

High-Fructose Corn Syrup (HFCS)

As if sugar wasn't bad enough already, they decided to start putting high-fructose corn syrup (HFCS) in all manner of beverages and foods. HFCS is cheaper and easier to manufacture than sucrose (table sugar), which explains why it has become so prevalent.

The problem is that excessive fructose consumption carries many risks, including contributing to insulin resistance and cardiovascular diseases.[48]

Fructose (which is fruit sugar) cannot be used by our body's cells for energy. It can only be metabolised in the liver, as a way to replenish its energy stores. However, once the liver's energy stores are topped up, any excess fructose coming in will most likely have to be stored as fat.

This makes excessive fructose consumption harmful. Apart from weight gain, high consumption of fructose can damage the liver, promote the growth of pathogenic bacteria, and has a myriad of other negative effects in the body.[48]

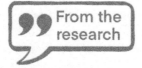

From the research

"Scientific data showed that fructose has the same effects on the liver as alcohol beverages which is already known as a liver toxin."[48]

Another little-known fact is that HFCS needs to be extracted in the presence of mercuric chloride[49]- a highly toxic and corrosive compound of mercury and chlorine. This means that HFCS always carries the high risk of being contaminated with mercuric chloride, making it even more harmful than it already is. Even small amounts of this toxin can be detrimental, and worse even, it can accumulate in the body over time.

Let me clarify something here. Fructose from moderate fruit consumption is not the same as guzzling down cola drinks, so do not worry about your child consuming fruit (as long as it is not in excess).

MSG

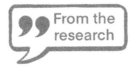

From the research

"The safety and toxicity of MSG had become controversial in the last few years because of reports of adverse reactions in people who have eaten foods that contain MSG. Many studies had confirmed the adverse reactions of MSG. MSG has been reported to cause headache, vomiting, diarrhea, irritable bowel syndrome, asthma attacks in asthmatic patients and panic attacks."[50]

Monosodium glutamate (MSG) is a common flavour enhancer that is used to give foods a savoury, broth-like taste, also called umami. MSG is added to soups, sauces, mixed condiments, chips, meat products, and puddings. Restaurant and take-away meals often carry the risk having MSG added to them. Chemicals like this are yet another reason to avoid processed or "ready-made" meals, and to be careful where you dine out.

MSG is an excitotoxin. That is to say, it can induce excitotoxicity. As you may remember from the last chapter, excitotoxicity can lead to neuronal cell damage or even cell death, which can, in turn, lead to neurodegeneration.

Though a controversial topic, with some saying MSG is completely safe and others arguing that it is toxic even in small quantities, the fact remains that some people do react badly to it and there have been reports of deleterious effects following ingestion.[45][50]

A lot of research has been done in animals and when taken together with adverse events reported in humans,[45][50] there is enough evidence to support the notion that food additives such as MSG are neither needed, nor wanted components in a healthy diet and lifestyle.

While occasional intake may be safe for adults in good health, for sensitive kids with health issues, it is best to keep it out of the diet.

This may prove to be more challenging than you would expect because MSG is often stealthily hidden in food under various cryptic names such as E621 or hydrolysed plant extract. We'll review some other names in Chapter Eight, so you're better equipped to steer clear of it.

Emulsifiers

Emulsifiers, also known as surfactants, are used to homogenise substances. For example, fat and water don't mix, but with an emulsifier you can create a smooth salad cream. Emulsifiers are widely used in the food industry where you'll find them in products such as:

- Baked goods
- Confectionery
- Dairy products
- Condiments such as ketchup and mayonnaise
- Oils, butter, and margarine
- Ice cream
- Beverages
- Chocolate
- Other "convenient" foods

Emulsifiers are also used in pharmaceuticals as absorption enhancers. In fact, in many cases the same ones used in medications are added to foods.[44]

Numerous synthetic emulsifiers have been shown to increase intestinal permeability and there is ample scientific evidence that these additives impair gut barrier function, even at the seemingly low concentrations used in industrial food processing.[44]

Certain emulsifiers that contain aluminium are approved for use in the food industry. One category of aluminium-containing emulsifiers is sodium aluminium phosphates (SALPs), which are one of the biggest contributors of aluminium to the diet.[51] They are commonly added to cheeses to improve texture, and slicing and melting properties. You will find SALPs in frozen pizzas, cookies, biscuits, muffins, cakes, and other baked goods.

Food Colourants

Artificial food colourings, many of which are made from petroleum, can bind to various human proteins in the gut or blood which, as you now know, can trigger a series of immune reactions that can lead to autoimmunity.[52]

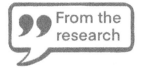

"Artificial food colorings, though known to cause DNA damage, adverse effects on the liver and kidneys, and have carcinogenic properties, have not been restricted. Instead, they have actually been increased in use for a growing number of foods over the last 50 years."[16]

Other negative effects that artificial food colourings can have include:[52]

- Causing hyperactivity in children
- Increase leaky gut
- Interfere with digestive enzymes
- Trigger immune responses to food
- Cause hypersensitivity to other toxins
- Cause or contribute to hay-fever and asthma
- Contribute to liver toxicity
- Contribute to mitochondrial dysfunction

Water Additives

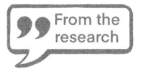

"Scientists have proven that there are more than 600 undesirable chemicals formed through the mutual action of water treatment disinfectants and contaminants in source water"[53]

Tap water has become polluted for several reasons:

- Many chemicals are added to municipal water supplies
- Human and industrial contamination (medications, antibiotics, petrol by-products, solvents)
- Agricultural runoff (herbicides, pesticides, artificial fertilisers, and many other chemicals)

Fluoride and chlorine are naturally occurring elements, but we'll discuss them here because they are used as additives to water, and by extension they make it into foods prepared with water.

Fluoride

Fluoride is added to the water in many places, including some US states and European countries. It's also used in toothpaste, mouthwash, dental treatments, pesticides, fertilisers, and even some foods and beverages.

Over 300 animal and human studies have shown that fluoride is toxic to brain and nervous system tissues. Numerous studies have found an association between lowered IQ in children and exposure to fluoride.[54] Fluoride can cause or contribute to:[20][55][56]

- Excitotoxicity
- Damage to cell membranes
- Depletion of glutathione and other antioxidants
- Inhibition of certain antioxidant enzymes (which enhances the toxicity of other chemicals)
- Inhibition of melatonin production
- Disruption of mitochondrial energy production enzymes
- Displaces iodine, which interferes with thyroid function

Aluminium and fluoride are harmful enough on their own, but in unison they can be even more so. The two can bind together to create a chemical complex that is toxic to neurons even at low concentrations. Fluoride also enhances aluminium absorption across the gut barrier and the blood-brain barrier.[20][55] Here you have a prime example of how toxic compounds can have an even greater effect when they act in synergy.

Chlorine

Chlorine is added to water as a disinfectant, to kill bacteria. After what you've learnt about the gut microbiota and its critical role in our health, do you think drinking chlorine would be good for your child's microbiota? You got it - it wouldn't be good.

Chlorine is associated with many disorders and exposure has even been linked to some cancers.[53] It doesn't just enter our bodies through drinking water. Because it is a volatile element, it readily evaporates from water, which means that we can inhale it when showering or sitting by the pool. It's even absorbed through the skin when we bathe or swim in chlorinated pools.

Common Pollutants in Household Products

There are countless chemicals polluting your home. We'll only review a few of them here for the sake of brevity, but I'll cover strategies to reduce your child's exposure to many more in Chapter Eight.

Phthalates

Phthalates are one of the most widespread toxic chemicals in our environment. They are used to make plastics soft and pliable and are added to many cosmetics and beauty products. We get exposed to phthalates through food, air, and skin contact. Some of the most common products where you'll find them include:

- PVC plastics
- Children's toys
- Plastic bags and some food packaging
- Cosmetics (e.g. perfumes, shampoo, nail polish, skin care products)
- Insecticides and insect repellents
- Building materials (e.g. paint, varnish)
- Detergents

Phthalates are anti-androgenic chemicals that can cause reproductive damage and alter sexual development in children. They disrupt the metabolism of the hormone testosterone, which is important for the development of boys. Phthalates can also interfere with thyroid hormone regulation.[57]

PVC floors are a common source of airborne phthalate dust. One study found that children who lived in homes with PVC flooring had higher rates of autism than those that lived in homes with wood flooring.[58]

Furthermore, another group of researchers found that mothers of autistic children had higher likelihood of exposure to canned foods, plastics, waste incinerators, old electronics, microwavable food, and printed fabrics than mothers of typically developing children.[59] Those products are sources of exposure to not just phthalates, but also toxins such as BPA and flame retardants.

Other studies have found higher levels of phthalates in the urine of autistic children than in their peers,[60][61] as well as reduced capacity to detoxify these compounds.[62]

As you can see, the dangers of phthalate exposure are real and pressing.

Bisphenol A (BPA)

BPA is a chemical that has been in use since the early 1960s to harden plastics. It is a hormonal disruptor that can induce oxidative stress and mitochondrial dysfunction.[57][63][64]

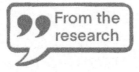

From the research

"The majority of children are exposed to bisphenol-A (BPA) through the use of plastic bottles and pacifiers."[16]

Studies have shown BPA levels to be higher in autistic children. Researchers who found BPA in the urine of autistic children at levels 15 times higher than the neurotypical controls concluded that there was an association between BPA exposure and ASD.[65]

BPA is found in many consumer products, including:

- Hard plastics
- Plastic bottles (including some baby bottles), cups, and containers
- Pacifiers
- Children's toys
- In some food packaging (e.g. lining of tin cans or juice boxes, even in some infant formula containers in the USA)

BPA and its metabolites can bind to various human proteins (including tissues in the brain) to form neo-antigens that the immune system marks for destruction. As you know, this is one way neuroautoimmunity and neurodegeneration can get triggered.[16]

Flame Retardants

Fire-retardant chemicals such as PBDEs (polybrominated diphenyl ethers) are found in:

- Furniture
- Beds
- Children's toys and clothing (e.g. pyjamas)
- Carpets
- Curtains
- Car seats
- Textiles
- Household appliances
- Electrical wiring
- Construction materials

Because they are used in so many products, PBDEs have now moved into our food chain. Levels have been found to be high in children (not just autistic children).[66]

Food, dust, and air are the main sources of exposure, but small children also get exposed to these chemicals via other vectors, including breastfeeding and through hand-to-mouth activities when playing.[66]

PBDEs and other similar chemicals are toxic to our cells at minute concentrations. They can cause significant damage to our mitochondria, oxidative stress, and can induce cell death. They even have the ability to cross the blood-brain barrier and bioaccumulate in our tissues.[1] Research has also shown that PBDEs can interfere with thyroid function.[67]

Formaldehyde

Formaldehyde is a highly reactive chemical, used in countless household products, and is a known carcinogen (cancer-causing agent). It, and its cousin glutaraldehyde, are common disinfecting chemicals that many of us are exposed to on a daily basis. Like many other harmful chemicals, formaldehyde can bind to human tissues and instigate immune responses via antibody production and subsequent immune activation, which can lead to autoimmunity.[16]

Common sources of exposure include:[68]

- Building materials and insulation
- Household products such as glues, permanent press fabrics, paints and coatings, lacquers and finishes, and paper products
- Preservatives used in some medicines, cosmetics and other consumer products, such as dishwashing liquids and fabric softeners.
- Fertilisers and pesticides
- Furniture
- Resins used in the manufacture of composite wood products

Furniture, mattresses, and carpets give off harmful compounds like formaldehyde for weeks, or even months, after you purchase them. In Chapter Eight, we'll consider some strategies to minimise the toxic effects of buying new furniture.

What Can You Do About It?

In Part Two of the *Autism Wellbeing Plan*, you will learn how to:

- Test for heavy metals and, when appropriate, for toxic chemicals (Chapter Six)
- Clean up your home from the major sources of exposure (Chapter Eight)
- Support your child's detoxification systems (Chapter Eleven and Twelve)

Wrap-up

This chapter concludes Part One of the book. You learnt the reasons children are more vulnerable to toxic insults than adults and the many ways in which harmful compounds can wreak havoc in our bodies.

We briefly looked at research linking heavy metals and autism severity before examining the most prevalent metals in our environment in more detail. As you saw, we are exposed to them from all angles - our air, water, food, and everyday products.

Finally, we looked at a few of the most common chemicals and additives in our food supply and environment.

The most important takeaways from this chapter are:

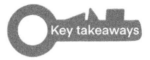

- Non-organic agriculture uses countless chemicals, some of which have been implicated in ASD and other conditions
- Processed foods are rife with harmful additives such as table salt, sweeteners, flavours, colours, and emulsifiers
- Tap water is contaminated with chemicals from industry, agriculture, and human activities
- Plastics and many household products are a source of invisible but nonetheless harmful chemical exposures

The good news (yes, there is good news) is that we will look at strategies you can use to reduce your family's toxic exposures significantly in Chapter Eight.

PART TWO - YOUR AUTISM WELLBEING PLAN

OVERVIEW OF PART TWO

Great work, you made it this far and I'm proud of you. I know that was a lot of information to take in, but you have equipped yourself with important knowledge that will evolve and develop over time. You'll see that it is empowering.

In a sense, though, we're only getting started. It's time to turn knowledge into action because that's where the rewards lie for you and your family.

As we discussed at the beginning of the Autism Wellbeing Plan, your child's health-building program will focus on diet, supplementation, reducing toxic exposure, sleep, and using lab testing to guide the process. In more detail, you will learn how to:

- Identify gut infections, metabolic imbalances, nutrient deficiencies, food sensitivities, and toxic exposures (Chapter Six)
- Implement a healthy gluten-free and casein-free diet, and remove potentially inflammatory foods and additives from your child's diet, while replacing them with healthy whole foods (**Chapter Seven** and **Eight**)
- Clean up your home to reduce chemical burden on your youngster (**Chapter Eight**)
- Improve the sleep environment and instil positive habits to promote restorative sleep (**Chapter Nine**)
- Support your child with the core five supplements (**Chapter Ten**)
- Use advanced supplementation strategies for specific situations or purposes (**Chapter Eleven**)

Finally, in **Chapter Twelve**, we will put everything you've learnt together. I will show you how to approach the design of your child's health-building program and give you an example of one, so you know what to expect when working with your practitioner.

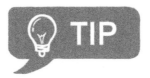

Now might be a good time to start thinking about how you will involve your child in this process. It is, after all, their journey to improved wellbeing that we are supporting. How you approach this will vary depending on their age, and needs, but you will know best.

As you read on, consider how you could make the process of collecting test samples, changing the diet and sleep routine, and taking supplements more like a game or mission, rather than a chore. Being open and honest is always the best policy - children are way too smart and perceptive for us to consider any other strategy.

With older children, you can explain the benefits that their improved health will bring (better sleep, less anxiety, less gut discomfort, more energy to play), while with younger kids you can use your creativity (involving the whole family in the new routines helps, as kids often like to follow suit).

Either way, I know you've got this.

Are you ready? Then let's get to it.

CHAPTER SIX: LAB TESTING TO IDENTIFY IMBALANCES AND HEALING OPPORTUNITIES

Overview of this Chapter

Every autistic child will have a unique and often complex case. In order to design the most personalised health-building program possible, you and your health care provider will need to utilise some laboratory (lab) tests. Thankfully, nowadays, we have many advanced tests where you can conveniently collect the sample at home, and have it picked up by a courier for shipping. It has never been easier to get the data you need to improve your child's wellbeing.

When we break down the lab testing you can do, we have three categories:

- Tests you run at the start of the health-building program
- Tests you use to monitor your child's progress allowing you to course-correct as required
- Specialised tests that you only run in certain circumstances

The foundational tests we'll cover shortly are:

- Organic acids test
- Stool pathogen screening
- Blood tests

- Food sensitivities testing
- Hair mineral analysis

Of course, you may not be able to run all the tests at once, or a couple may not yet be needed. We'll tackle different scenarios, and prudent ways to proceed in this chapter and Chapter Twelve.

When your practitioner recommends it, you may want to run some more specialised tests. My initial intent was to include a wide variety of advanced tests in the *Autism Wellbeing Plan*. However, I decided to give you an overview in this chapter and put the bulk of the information online for these reasons:

- You've had more than enough information to digest and probably won't want to be inundated with more cryptic names and biomarkers.
- In many cases, the foundational tests would provide most of the clinical value.
- I'll show you how to spot clues that more advanced testing may be needed, at which time the information will be there for you online.

After reviewing the foundational tests, we'll briefly look into:

- Other ways to test for heavy metals and essential minerals
- Mycotoxin testing (for mould toxins)
- Chemical toxicity testing
- Tests for autoimmunity

Links to all the tests discussed in this chapter will be on the book's resources webpage. Let me stress this: I have no affiliation with any of the labs whose tests I recommend. My recommendations are based solely on the value the tests provide, and there are no profit or marketing motives involved.

The Importance of Testing for Pathogens

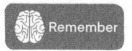

It bears repeating again and again: testing for pathogens is probably the most important thing you need to do when it comes to improving your child's health. Many stubborn infections or overgrowths won't just resolve themselves, even with improved diet, probiotics, and other supplement support. You need to identify and address any offending organisms as a matter of priority.

You also need to be aware that challenges exist when testing for pathogens. Certain tests have limitations, and some are better than others. Often, a complementary approach to testing is the best choice. However, not every family will have the insurance coverage or funds to run the optimal test recommendations, so we'll look at the various options you have.

In a nutshell, here's how to go about it, depending on your current level of resources:

- **If you have no insurance coverage and can only afford one test:** run the organic acids test (OAT).
- **If you can afford it or have the insurance coverage:** run the OAT and a comprehensive stool pathogen screening.
- **If you have insurance but the OAT is not covered by it:** get whatever stool test you can for free and run the OAT if you can afford it. Otherwise, use whatever testing is covered by your insurance.

Why would I recommend that you run both an OAT and a stool test, if possible? The reason is that both types of test are good at detecting different organisms.

For example, the OAT (which is a urine test) is great at detecting *Candida* and *Clostridia*. However, *Candida* is difficult to grow in a petri dish, so it's often missed on stool tests. Likewise, *Clostridium difficile*'s toxins are sometimes not detected in stool specimens.

On the other hand, stool tests can detect many pathogens that are not specifically tested for by the OAT, such as parasites, worms, protozoa, and sometimes certain viruses. Some stool tests have the added advantage of screening our beneficial bacteria and markers for digestive health, which can help your clinician build a better picture of the state of your child's gut.

Organic Acids Test

The organic acids test (OAT) is the most useful test you can run for your child, especially at the beginning of their health-building program. Organic acids are metabolic by-products that are representative of our metabolism's functions. We can measure them in urine, which makes the OAT sample easy to collect at home and the test non-invasive. This takes much stress off your child as driving to the clinic, waiting, and getting a blood-draw can be an uncomfortable experience.

There are several labs offering organic acids testing. My personal recommendation would be to use the one from the Great Plains Laboratory (GPL) because of how comprehensive their panel is. When talking about organic acids testing, I'll be referring to the GPL panel, but many of the markers they test for would be included on other OAT panels.

The GPL OAT provides a comprehensive snapshot of a person's metabolic function and overall health. It includes about 75 markers for urinary metabolites, which test the following areas:

- Yeast and fungal overgrowths
- Bacterial markers, including *Clostridia* overgrowth
- Neurotransmitter metabolism
- Nutrient status
- Antioxidant (glutathione) status
- Oxalate metabolites
- Glucose and fatty acid metabolism (some of these markers can be helpful in identifying mitochondrial dysfunction)
- Amino acid metabolites

I'll discuss the sections most relevant to ASD below.

Yeast and Fungal Markers

As you know, yeast overgrowth is very common in autistic children. The OAT provides several useful markers which can indicate the presence of *Candida*, as well as *Aspergillus* and other fungal species and their toxic by-products.

When certain markers on the OAT are elevated, it's a strong indication for mould toxicity. In those instances, testing for mycotoxins is a good idea. I'll show you the specific markers in Chapter Twelve.

Bacterial Markers

The OAT includes several bacterial markers that can indicate a state of general dysbiosis in your child's gut. The panel also includes markers for *Clostridia* bacteria. As I mentioned earlier, *Clostridia* are sometimes missed on stool tests, which makes the OAT particularly valuable clinically.

Nutritional Markers

The GPL OAT panel tests the status of the following nutrients:

- Vitamin B_2
- Vitamin B_5
- Vitamin B_6
- Vitamin B_{12}
- Vitamin C
- Biotin
- Coenzyme Q_{10}
- N-acetylcysteine (NAC)

These are functional nutrient markers and may be even more useful for evaluating your child's nutrient status than blood testing. This is because the body buffers the blood to quite tight physiological ranges, often at the expense of its tissues and organs. So, a blood test may come back within the lab range, but the status of the nutrient may be far from healthy or optimal.

In fact, if a blood marker is so out of range that your doctor decides to do something about it, it's often very late in the process. You want to catch functional or sub-clinical deficiencies early so that you can correct them before problems start occurring.

Indicators of Detoxification

The OAT has two markers that, when elevated, can indicate a glutathione deficiency. As you now know, glutathione levels can be depleted due to oxidative stress, heavy metal and chemical toxicity, gut infections, or other stressors.

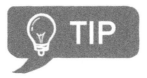

A low glutathione status usually indicates that you need to identify and reduce the factors contributing to its depletion and support your child with antioxidants.

Neurotransmitter Metabolism

The OAT has several markers for metabolites of important neurotransmitters such as:

- Dopamine
- Norepinephrine/epinephrine (noradrenaline/adrenalin)
- Serotonin

Dysregulated neurotransmitter metabolism can have wide-ranging effects on behaviour, mood, sleep, and cognition. Catching imbalances as soon as possible is imperative.

The markers on the OAT can be low or elevated due to many reasons, such as:

- Genetic variations or disorders
- Nutrient deficiencies
- Gut infections (e.g. *Clostridia*)
- Medications or supplements
- Toxic exposure
- Certain foods can cause elevations

Oxalate Metabolites

The GPL OAT is the only commercially available test on the market that evaluates levels of oxalate in urine. It includes three oxalate markers, two of which may indicate a genetic disorder in oxalate metabolism.

Mitochondrial Markers

The OAT has multiple markers that can indicate the presence of mitochondrial dysfunction. We will review the most useful ones in Chapter Twelve.

Stool Pathogen Testing

Not all stool tests are created equal. If you're going to invest the time and money to run one, you're best off using a reputable lab. For an up-to-date list of stool tests from quality labs, visit the resources webpage for this book.

Traditional stool tests are culture-based. This means that the organisms are grown, or cultured, in petri dishes. After several days, a lab technician inspects the sample, and some automated tests may be run, depending on the lab.

Some limitations of culture-based stool tests include:

- Certain bacteria and yeasts are difficult or impossible to culture (e.g. anaerobic bacteria that thrive in environments without oxygen)
- Manually inspecting a sample by a lab technician is an error-prone process
- Higher chance of "false negatives" (when the person is infected with the organism, but the test comes back as negative)
- Some labs require two or three stool samples to be collected, which can be inconvenient

A more recent type of test is the DNA-based stool test, where the genetic material of the organisms is analysed to identify them. The advantages of this type of test include:

- Requires only one stool sample
- Higher accuracy
- Test is automated, so less error-prone
- Usually a faster turnaround time than culture-based tests
- They allow the identification of up to 50% of organisms that may be have been missed by culture techniques.[1]

One potential issue with DNA-based stool tests is that they have a higher chance of "false positives". You may see many more organisms detected, but not all of them will necessarily be causing your child distress. A skilled clinician should take your unique case into consideration and won't over-interpret the test results.

My personal preference is to use the DNA-based test if possible, as it's more convenient to collect just one sample and because of the reduced chances of missing some organisms. However, there are several labs that excel at culture-based tests, so they are great alternatives, especially when your insurance covers them but not a DNA-based test (or it is not available to you). Remember that I have some links on the resources webpage if you want to do further research.

Blood Tests

It's important to get a baseline of data at the start of your child's health-building program. You want to identify any glaring imbalances quickly so you may begin to address them. Your health care provider should run an initial set of labs that, at the least, includes the following markers:

- Complete blood count (CBC)
- Comprehensive metabolic panel
- Zinc (in plasma)
- Copper (in serum)
- Iron and ferritin
- Folate and vitamin B_{12}
- Vitamin D
- Blood lipids (cholesterol, HDL, LDL)
- Thyroid panel (TSH, T3, T4)
- Homocysteine
- C-reactive protein (hs-CRP)

The above are standard tests, so you should be able to get them through your doctor in most cases. Depending on your insurance coverage, they may even be free.

If anything comes back out of the ordinary, you will want to run repeat tests periodically to make sure the program is correcting any imbalances.

For example, let's say homocysteine, a marker for inflammation, comes back high. Your practitioner recommends starting to supplement your child with vitamin B_{12} and folate. After 8-12 weeks, you would want to check the homocysteine value again to see if supplementation is helping to lower it, which is a sign that the methylation cycle is running more smoothly than it was before. If the homocysteine is still high, your practitioner may recommend increasing the vitamin B_{12} and folate, or they may add TMG to the program. (We will talk more about these and other supplements in Chapter Eleven.)

Testing Zinc and Copper Status

It's worth covering testing for zinc and copper in more depth, because it's so crucial to address an imbalance in these minerals. As mentioned in Chapter Four, this is the most common imbalance in autistic children, and it has even been associated with ASD severity in some studies. You don't want to skip this test.

The basic zinc and copper blood work is inexpensive, and you might even get it done for free. The best markers to use are plasma zinc[2] and serum copper.

An ideal plasma zinc to serum copper ratio is about 1:1, though the optimal blood range is 0.70 to 1.00 of zinc to copper.[3]

You get the ratio by dividing the zinc value on the test by the copper value. The lower the ratio gets, the more severe the zinc-copper imbalance becomes. Ratios as low as ~0.61 have been reported in ASD studies.[3][4] I've seen even lower.

Food Sensitivities Testing

The gold standard for identifying food sensitivities is the elimination diet, followed by a provocation test. Simply put, you remove the food from your child's diet for a period of time (e.g. 3 to 6 months), then have them eat it and monitor for reactions. With older children, you can have them give you their input on how the food makes them feel.

If you have the time and energy, you can certainly try this with some foods (especially if you have a hunch that your child may be reacting to them). But you're probably thinking that it sounds like a massive hassle to do with the entire diet, especially with younger kids. I don't blame you. Rotating and keeping track of foods is a cumbersome process, especially when the rest of the family continues to eat the foods you want to exclude from your child's diet.

This is where a food sensitivities panel can come in handy. In this section, I'll introduce you to the topic by giving you an overview of:

- IgG Testing (the most common type of test)
- The Mediator Release Test (MRT) and the value it offers
- Several more specialised tests available on the market

Let me preface the discussion by telling you that testing for food sensitivities is not as straightforward as you might think (or practitioners would like it to be). Whereas food allergies are relatively simple to test for (IgE antibodies), food sensitivities are much more complex and involve many mechanisms of the innate and adaptive immune systems.

The first issue is that labs usually test for raw foods, which may give us misleading results because cooking proteins changes them. We also tend to combine foods into meals, which further complicates matters because food proteins in combination can cause stronger immune reactions in some people.[5-7]

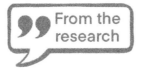
From the research

"One of the biggest problems with food immune reactivity tests is that the foods used in the panels do not reflect the manner in which the patient consumes the food. Research has shown that heating food above 118°F changes the protein structure, which changes the antigenicity of the food."[5]

A further confounding variable is that the antigens used in tests may be different across labs, or in some cases contaminated with bacteria, fungi, metals, or pesticides. This means you could get different results from different labs, or sometimes even from the same lab!

Additionally, some labs measure antibodies at the protein level, while others measure them at the peptide level. Measuring at the peptide level is like using a magnifying glass to scan for finer details on a picture. This method offers more accuracy and specificity, but is more expensive.

So, what do you do? Here's my advice:

- Know when it's worth doing the test and when it isn't the right time (I'll cover the most common scenarios in Chapter Twelve).
- Always go with a reputable lab (there are links to a few on the resources webpage). Some labs test samples up to three times to ensure the accuracy of the results. That's the kind of quality standards you need to look for.
- Do not over-interpret or rely on the test results too much. For example, a food may come back as non-reactive, but your child clearly reacts to it. In such cases, you need to use your own judgement and keep the food out of the diet.
- Similarly, you need to remain vigilant. Food sensitivities develop and change over time, so you need to continue monitoring your child's reactions and catch any anomalies.

With that said, let's move onto our discussion of the tests available to you.

IgG Testing

IgG (immunoglobulin G) tests measure the levels of IgG antibodies in the person's blood to various foods. Depending on the panel you choose, they can include as many as 180 different foods including meat, seafood, dairy, fruits, vegetables, grains, nuts, seeds, and herbs.

The advantage of this type of test is that they are more cost-effective than the others we'll discuss (quality panels as low as $150 are available) and they can provide useful information that you can use to refine your child's diet.

The important caveat is that your child must be consuming the foods to get an accurate representation of reactivity. When you don't eat a certain food, the body gradually stops producing antibodies to it. That is essentially the purpose of eliminating reactive foods from the diet. It gives the immune system a break. In the meantime, hopefully, any underlying gut (or other) issues contributing to the sensitivity are addressed.

Now, this is not to say if your child is on a gluten-free diet that you now need to start them back on gluten to see if they react to it. What it means is that if your child doesn't eat certain foods for several months, they won't be producing IgG antibodies to them, and the test cannot tell you whether they are problematic.

A disadvantage of most IgG tests is they don't test for the various "parts" of dairy and wheat proteins. Rather, they look at the whole food (though some labs now offer more in-depth testing).

So, a test may show that milk or wheat are non-reactive, but that does not necessarily mean that some little protein in these foods isn't triggering your child's immune system. In fact, studies have shown that it's not just autistic children that react to various wheat and milk proteins, but also healthy blood donors.[5][8] We'll revisit the topic of wheat and milk, and the potential problems they can cause in the next chapter.

Finally, keep in mind that IgG antibodies is only one way a person can react to foods. Other antibodies (IgA, IgM) or non-antibody responses may also play a role in food sensitivities, but these won't be detected on this type of test. That's why I said it's important to not be overly reliant on any test result.

In summary, you need to know when an IgG test will provide value, and when to skip it. As mentioned, we'll discuss the various ways to go about it in Chapter Twelve.

The Mediator Release Test (MRT)

One very useful test I would recommend is the Mediator Release Test (MRT) from Oxford Biomedical Technologies Inc. The lab exposes your child's blood to various foods and food additives, then measures the immune response to each of them. The higher the immune response, the more likely that the food will be reactive for them. The beauty of this approach is that your child doesn't need to be eating the foods prior to running the test.

The MRT is one of the best tests to use if you want to expand your child's diet but want to minimise the foods to which they are likely to react.

At this time, the panel is available in the US, UK, and EU, and you have the option to analyse 85, 130, or 170 foods and chemicals.

Another thing I like about the MRT is that it measures reactivity to common food additives, preservatives, sweeteners, and medications, such as:

- Aspartame
- Fructose (High-fructose corn syrup)
- MSG
- Various food colourants
- Ibuprofen
- Lecithin (soy)
- Potassium nitrate
- Salicylic acid
- Polysorbate 80
- Saccharin
- Tyramine
- Benzoic acid
- Acetaminophen

More Specialised Tests

Over the past decade, more advanced food sensitivities panels have come to the market. Some labs now offer:

- Testing for more than just IgG antibodies (e.g. IgA)
- Comprehensive analysis of reactivity to the various proteins in gluten and non-gluten wheat proteins
- Detection of antibodies that indicate the presence of leaky gut
- Panels that test for cooked and raw foods (not cheap, mind you)

When would you run a more advanced panel?

- You want to make sure your child reacts to gluten or milk before you decide to implement the gluten-free, casein-free (GFCF) diet
- You have implemented the GFCF and now you want to ensure your child is not reacting to newly introduced foods, or to foods that are commonly over-consumed on the GFCF diet (e.g. amaranth, buckwheat, millet, potatoes, rice, sorghum, or quinoa)
- You have the resources to pay for the test or your insurance covers it

In case you're curious, here are some examples of advanced panels from reputable labs:

- Vibrant Wellness – Wheat Zoomer
- Cyrex Laboratories' Array #3X - Wheat/Gluten Proteome Reactivity & Autoimmunity
- Cyrex Laboratories' Array #4 - Gluten-Associated Cross-Reactive Foods and Foods Sensitivity

For the most up-to-date list of specialised panels, please visit the resources webpage for the book.

Hair Mineral Analysis

Hair Tissue Mineral Analysis (HMA) is a useful and inexpensive test that has multiple purposes, including to:

- Detect toxic metals being excreted
- Check status of essential minerals and detect inadequate nutritional status of certain ones
- Monitor copper excretion when balancing zinc and copper levels

Many clinicians and researchers use HMA to analyse levels of nutrient minerals and toxic metals in autistic children.[9-13] I've cited some research in various parts of the book.

Hair is an excretory tissue. This means that HMA cannot be used on its own to detect acute heavy metal toxicity or mineral deficiencies. Nor can it be used as a gauge for your child's current body burden of toxic metals.

Rather, hair testing provides a historical snapshot. Hair grows at about 1cm (0.4in) per month, so a 3cm (1.2in) sample gives us about three months of data. We use HMA to see which heavy metals your child has been excreting over the past 2-3 months, as well as to monitor longer-term mineral status.

HMA samples are easy to collect and stable (much more so than urine, stool, or blood samples). The non-invasive nature of this type of test makes it especially convenient.

Monitoring Essential Minerals with HMA

Not every mineral in hair directly corresponds with the body's level of that mineral. Minerals that *do* correlate with levels in the body include:[14]

- Zinc
- Copper
- Magnesium
- Selenium
- Chromium

Luckily, these are some of the most interesting minerals to us. Occasionally, you may want a more comprehensive analysis of your child's essential mineral status, such as at the start of their health-building program, or during chelation therapy. In those cases, blood testing can provide you with the data you need.

More Advanced Testing

As I mentioned at the start of this chapter, the resources webpage for this book contains up-to-date links to the labs and tests that we discuss here. I will add more over time, so it's worth checking in occasionally. We'll now briefly look into:

- Other ways to test for heavy metals and essential minerals
- Mycotoxin testing (for mould toxins)
- Chemical toxicity testing
- Tests for autoimmunity

Testing for Heavy Metals and Essential Minerals

Hair mineral analysis is useful when designing a standard health-building protocol, but your practitioner may sometimes recommend additional tests.

The various methods of assessing a person's levels of metals and minerals cover different time-ranges. Briefly, they are:

- **Urine:** a measure of recent exposure (several days)[15]
- **Red blood cells (RBC) analysis:** measures longer term mineral status and recent or ongoing exposure to toxic metals
- **Whole blood analysis:** an intermediate between urine and RBC analysis[15]

- **Hair mineral analysis:** gives us a picture of longer term mineral status and excretion of toxic metals (months)

Let's take a brief look at urine and blood testing, and when you may use them.

Urine Testing

Urine tests are often used during chelation (metal detoxification) therapy to monitor the effectiveness of the chelating (metal-binding) agents used (e.g. DMSA, DMPS, and EDTA). I'll briefly discuss chelation in Chapter Twelve.

The urine sample usually requires the collection of all urine in a 24-hour period, after which a small sample is taken and sent to the lab. You can probably imagine this makes the process quite cumbersome and error-prone, especially with smaller children.

You probably won't need to use this type of test in most cases, unless your practitioner recommends chelation or decides to run it because they suspect your child has had recent exposure to heavy metals.

Blood Testing

Blood testing of minerals and metals can be done in three ways:

- In plasma
- Red blood cell (RBC) analysis
- Whole blood analysis (measures plasma and RBC)

The most commonly used methods are RBC and whole blood analysis. RBC analysis is one of the best ways to check your child's essential mineral status, though whole blood analysis can also be used to detect nutrient mineral inadequacies or imbalances.

When it comes to toxic metals, RBC and whole blood testing can be used as an indication of recent or ongoing exposure, but cannot be used to gauge your child's body burden of the metals. These tests are also often used before starting chelation therapy, as well as during its course to monitor the child's mineral status and level of toxic metal excretion.

The major downside of blood tests is, of course, that they require a blood draw, which can be challenging or traumatising for some kids. They are usually more expensive than HMA and urine analysis.

The primary advantage of blood tests is that they give you data on your child's current mineral levels. You can't get this information with a hair test and it may be useful in identifying mineral deficiencies or inadequacies.

Why didn't I include them in the foundational tests, then? My reasoning is:

- We already know that autistic children's nutrient status is likely to be suboptimal.
- The basic blood tests cover zinc, copper, and iron, which are of particular interest to us.
- No matter your child's nutrient status, you are still going to need to support them with vitamins and minerals long-term.
- The diet, supplementation, and other recommendations in the book will address many nutrient inadequacies.

Having said that, a comprehensive blood mineral analysis can be extremely helpful when it identifies serious nutrient deficiencies.

So, while the extra cost may not always be justified, if you're covered by insurance or can afford it, having your child's nutrient status analysed at the start of their health-building program can help your practitioner design a better protocol. Also, monitoring with the occasional retest may be warranted in cases where the initial analysis found many deficiencies or inadequacies.

Mycotoxin Testing

In most cases, a comprehensive stool screening and the organic acids test will provide more than enough information for you and your practitioner to start improving your child's health.

Occasionally though, testing for mould toxins may be appropriate. As discussed in Chapter Three, mycotoxins are produced by certain types of moulds that can grow on food and in buildings.

There are several scenarios where I would recommend testing for mycotoxins:

- Your home has been water damaged in the past or shows signs of mould accumulation
- Your home has poor ventilation and damp areas conducive to mould growth
- Your child eats foods that are at risk for mould contamination (e.g. peanuts, corn, and other grains)

- The stool pathogen test comes back negative, but your child has gastrointestinal issues or other symptoms which we'll discuss in Chapter Twelve
- When certain markers on the organic acids test are elevated, it's a big clue that mycotoxins may be an issue for your child (I will go over these markers in Chapter Twelve)

The best way to test your child for mycotoxins is by running the Great Plains Laboratory's MycoTOX profile. Like the organic acids test, you can take the small urine sample at home and send it to the lab for analysis. You can even have the lab run both tests on the same sample, which is more economical.

The MycoTOX test screens for eleven mycotoxins that are produced by 40 species of mould, and so far, I haven't been able to find a test on the market that offers anywhere near the same value for money and quality.

Chemical Toxicity Testing

Awareness of toxic exposures is the first step in actually doing something about them. If you suspect your child may have recent or chronic exposure, a chemical toxicity test can confirm it and tell you which chemicals are involved. This can help you identify the source and work to eliminate it. It can also signal that your child may need extra nutritional support for their detoxification systems.

We will look at two tests that are different in terms of what they can detect, but both can be useful at the right time.

Great Plains Laboratory's GPL-TOX

One of the best tests for chemical exposure is the Great Plains Laboratory's GPL-TOX. It tests for 172 different environmental pollutants using 18 different metabolites. A single urine sample is taken at home and sent to the lab for analysis. Similar to the MycoTOX profile, you can combine this test with the organic acids test and only have to send in one sample. The GPL-TOX tests for the following chemicals:

- Phthalates (we discussed their prevalence in Chapter Five)
- Vinyl chloride (sources may include materials made with PVC)
- Benzene

- Pyrethrins (in insecticides)
- Xylenes (in paint, varnish, pesticides, cleaning fluids, exhaust fumes, perfumes)
- Styrene (used in plastics manufacture, food packaging)
- Organophosphates (pesticides)
- 2,4-dichlorophenoxyacetic (2,4-D) (used in agriculture, herbicides, on genetically modified crops)
- MTBE and ETBE (petrol additives, may contaminate groundwater)
- Diphenyl phosphate (flame retardants used in plastics, electronic devices, some cosmetics)
- Others including acrylamide, perchlorate, 1,3 butadiene, propylene oxide, 1-bromopropane (1-BP), ethylene oxide, acrylonitrile

The GPL-TOX also has the marker tiglylglycine, which is a marker for mitochondrial dysfunction. Since many toxic chemicals target the mitochondria, this marker can be useful in ascertaining whether your child's mitochondria are being affected. We'll delve into this topic in more detail in Chapter Twelve.

Cyrex Laboratories' Array #11

Cyrex Laboratories' Array #11 is different from the GPL-TOX test, in that it tests for immune reactivity to various toxins (including several metals).

In other words, the lab measures levels of antibodies to heavy metals and chemicals, rather than the levels of the compounds themselves. This way, your clinician can build a picture of what particular chemicals or metals have bound themselves to your child's tissues and have become a body burden, causing the immune system to react to them.

So, while a heavy metal (e.g. hair analysis) or chemical test (like the GPL-TOX) can show *what* toxins your child has been exposed to, a test like this is useful in determining *which* of them are causing your child problems.

The Cyrex Array #11 measures various antibodies (IgA, IgG, or IgM) to the following toxins:

- Aflatoxins (mycotoxins produced by certain moulds, discussed in Chapter Three)
- Formaldehyde and glutaraldehyde (I briefly discussed these in Chapter Five)
- Bisphenol A and (also discussed in Chapter Five)

- Tetrabromobisphenol A (one of the most common flame retardants)
- Parabens (preservatives used in cosmetics and medications)
- Mercury compounds and other metals (nickel, cobalt, cadmium, lead, arsenic)
- Other hazardous substances such as isocyanate, trimellitic and phthalic anhydrides, benzene ring compounds, BPA binding protein, and tetrachloroethylene

This test is available in the US and Canada.

Testing for Autoimmune Antibodies

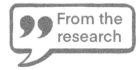

From the research

"When the target of autoantibodies is neurological tissues, the result will be neurodegeneration that can manifest as behavioral problems, movement disorders and communication difficulties seen in ASD."[16]

The subject of autoimmunity as it relates to ASD is gaining traction, but we're still far from a concrete understanding of all the mechanisms at play. There certainly seems to be a subset of children at higher risk.

In Chapter Two, you learnt that a disrupted gut could lead to a chain of events that can eventually lead to autoimmune reactions within the body. Because every person is so unique, how they will be affected by autoimmunity will differ greatly.

Your practitioner needs to take many variables into consideration before they recommend some more advanced tests.

Here is one simple way I would approach the situation. If any of the following apply to your child, it would support the case for testing for autoimmune antibodies:

- You have a family history of autoimmune disorders.
- Your child has signs of considerable immune system dysregu-

lation (e.g. allergies, severe food reactions, high levels of toxicity, leaky gut, gut infections).

- You notice a sudden change or worsening of neurological symptoms.

One of the most basic autoimmunity tests you can run is the antinuclear antibodies (ANA) test. It screens for antibodies that target parts of the cell's nucleus. The test is cheap to run (I've seen it as low as $36 to order online) and if results are positive, it may prompt your clinician to run a more advanced autoimmunity panel. From there, you can start delving deeper into the matter.

There are specialised tests on the market that test for various antibodies to proteins in the human body. Some panels focus on neural tissues (brain and central nervous system), while more comprehensive ones include tissues from other systems and organs of the body (e.g. gut, liver, thyroid). To begin with, a test for neurological (brain) tissues would offer the most value.

Other than the ANA antibodies I mentioned above, studies have identified antibodies to the following neural proteins or structures in autistic children:[16-19]

- Blood-brain barrier proteins (s100b, glial fibrillary acidic protein)
- Purkinje cells
- Myelin basic protein (MBP)
- Myelin-associated glycoprotein (MAG)
- Myelin oligodendrocyte glycoprotein (MOG)
- Cerebellar
- Synapsin

So, when looking for a panel to run, your practitioner needs to recommend one that includes the above markers, at the very least.

The following panels are from reputable labs and screen for the above, and other autoimmune antibodies:

- Vibrant Wellness - Neural Zoomer and Neural Zoomer Plus
- Cyrex Laboratories' Array #7 - Neurological Autoimmune Reactivity Screen
- Cyrex Laboratories' Array #5 - Multiple Autoimmune Reactivity Screen

Rather than inundate you with more information, I have further links and resources on the above tests on the resources webpage. If you ever need to research this further, the information is there for you.

Wrap-up

In this chapter, I introduced you to the foundational tests you and your practitioner can use to inform the design of a truly customised health-building program for your child:

- Organic acids test
- Stool pathogen screening
- Blood tests
- Food sensitivities testing
- Hair mineral analysis

First, I emphasised the importance of testing your child for gut pathogens. It won't be the last time, either. That's how crucial it is.

Then we looked at the organic acids test (OAT) in more detail. Though we only covered areas most relevant to ASD, you saw how comprehensive and valuable the OAT can be in identifying metabolic imbalances and healing opportunities. There are many layers to the test that a skilled clinician will be able to leverage, which is why I recommend running it so strongly.

I discussed some limitations and advantages of stool pathogen screening methodologies, so you can make better decisions when you choose to run this type of test. We will revisit the topic of testing for gut bugs and protocols to support pathogen eradication in Chapter Twelve.

You learnt the basic blood tests you need to have your doctor run to identify potential imbalances, deficiencies, or inflammation. We took a deeper look at testing your child's zinc and copper balance.

Then I covered the fundamentals of food sensitivity testing. We delved into considerations around using the common IgG test, and I introduced you to the Mediator Release Test. You also learnt about more specialised panels and scenarios in which you may want to run them.

We wrapped up the foundational tests with hair mineral analysis and how you can use it to monitor your child's mineral status and the excretion of heavy metals and copper.

Finally, I introduced you to some more advanced tests and situations in which you may want to consider running them. We reviewed testing for:

- Heavy metals and essential minerals
- Mycotoxins
- Chemical exposure
- Autoimmune antibodies

In Chapter Twelve, I'll show you which markers on the organic acids test may indicate that testing for mycotoxins or chemical exposure is prudent.

While I could have filled half a book with other lab tests and descriptions, you will probably agree that what we covered is more than enough to get started. When you're ready for more information, be sure to check out the book's webpage for more links, videos, and other resources related to lab testing.

We will now switch gears and turn our attention to the practical aspects of your child's health-building program. The next topic we need to tackle is the most important aspect of your child's wellbeing - their diet.

CHAPTER SEVEN: DIET - THE HEALTHY GLU-TEN-FREE/CASEIN-FREE FOUNDATION

Overview of this Chapter

The most critical component of any health improvement program is the diet. You can think of it as the foundation of your house. It needs to be solid to hold the structure up, but it also needs to be free from cracks that can turn into a bigger problem down the line.

What cracks can your child's diet have? We often think we have it figured out - eat plenty of fruits and vegetables, some meat, and not too many sugary snacks or junk foods. But as you saw in Chapter Five, it's not so cut and dry.

To design a truly optimal diet to support health, we need to consider not just what foods to eat, but how those foods have been grown and processed.

We can't stop there, either. You might know the old saying by the Roman poet and philosopher Lucretius, "One man's meat is another man's poison." (Of course, in today's world he probably would have said "One person's meat, or plant-based substitute, is another person's poison.") What this means is, what's good for you might not be good for your child. Simple example: a supposedly healthy food, like spinach, may actually be doing them harm if their gut is leaky and oxalates are an issue (spinach is very high in oxalates).

Additionally, if you don't factor in food sensitivities or intolerances, your child may continue to eat foods that "should" be healthy but are instead causing inflammation and immune reactions.

So in actuality, doing the healthy diet thing in our day and age is a minefield. But I will show you how to navigate this minefield and come out on the other side unscathed.

In this chapter, we'll discuss the benefits and practical aspects of using the gluten-free and casein-free diet in your child's health-building program. I'll do my best to clear up some misconceptions about the diet and explain why gluten and the milk protein casein can become problematic for your child.

We'll also take a brief look at several more advanced diets and situations in which you may consider implementing them in your child's program.

As with other chapters, there will be further resources on the book's webpage.

The Power of Nutrients

What can a good diet and supplementation program do, really?

A lot.

More than you might think, in fact. Pretty much any disorder or (non-terminal) disease will improve when the person improves their diet and supplements it intelligently.

But let's not speculate. Can we look to any research for some evidence? Yes, we can. This has been part of my mission to ensure you have the right information backed up by solid research to give you the confidence that the suggestions in this book are valid and, more importantly, essential in helping you improve your child's quality of life.

A paper was published in 2018, which outlined a 12-month treatment study of a comprehensive nutritional and dietary program for autistic individuals of various ages. The program consisted of:[1]

- A multivitamin and mineral supplement
- Essential fatty acids
- Epsom salt baths
- Carnitine
- Digestive enzymes
- A healthy gluten-free, casein-free, soy-free (HGCSF) diet

Doesn't look too complex, does it? I would say many people might even dismiss a program like that, thinking that it is too simple to do much good in a condition as complex as ASD. But they would be wrong. Here is a quote from the authors of the study:

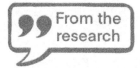

"The positive results of this study suggest that a comprehensive nutritional and dietary intervention is effective at improving nutritional status, non-verbal IQ, autism symptoms, and other symptoms in most individuals with ASD. Parents reported that the vitamin/mineral supplements, essential fatty acids, and HGCSF diet were the most beneficial."[1]

Not only did the group that received the treatment have their nutritional status improve measurably, their non-verbal intellectual ability improved significantly when compared to the non-treatment group of the study (autistic participants who did not follow a diet and supplement program).

The researchers reported that, based on the various assessments conducted, the individuals in the treatment group had significantly "greater improvement in autism symptoms and developmental age". Not bad for a few supplements and some dietary changes, right? That's before we even consider any improvements in general health the participants may have attained.

Various rating scales and assessment tools were used to evaluate the changes in the treatment and non-treatment groups. We won't discuss them here, but I'll leave you with the below quote before we move on. (This paper is available for free online and I would recommend you give it a read. It's quite readable for a scientific publication and has many finer details that we don't have space to cover here.)

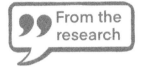

"During the 12 months of treatment, the non-treatment group gained only 4 months of development on the VABS-II, consistent with a major developmental delay. In contrast, the treatment group gained an average of 18 months of development, with substantial improvements in many areas. However, their average developmental age still remained well below their biological age, so that they were still significantly impaired. This is consistent with modest but significant improvements on the CARS-2 and SAS-Pro."[1]

In other words, the group that did the program gained 18 months of development in 12 months, while the non-treatment group gained only 4 months in that same time period. That alone should inspire every family to implement a comprehensive nutritional and supplementation program for their child. The earlier, the better.

Principles of a Healthy Diet

The core principles of a healthy diet for your child are:

- Organically grown fruits and vegetables
- Grass-fed meat, and pastured eggs and dairy products
- Wild-caught small fish (no farmed fish or large ocean fish)
- Clean, filtered water, free of contaminants
- Minimum possible processed or junk foods (free from sugar, artificial colours, additives, herbicides, pesticides and other chemicals)
- Exclude foods to which your child is allergic or sensitive
- Adequate calories - not too much or too little

After reading Chapter Five, you should now understand the importance of keeping the diet as clean as possible. If you follow the above principles as strictly as possible, you would be doing a tremendous service to your child. You might even be surprised how much their health improves in a short period of time.

The Role of the GFCF in Your Child's Health-Building Program

The goal of this chapter is not to sell you the gluten-free, casein-free (GFCF) diet as the "be-all, end-all" solution to anything. That's not the point of the GFCF diet at all. It is simply a steppingstone to getting your child as healthy as you can. It's a tool in your arsenal, to be utilised for as long as it is useful.

So, no matter what you've heard about the GFCF diet or what your preconceived notions are, please cast them aside while I do my best to show that there is value in giving it a proper trial.

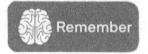

Let me re-iterate: the GFCF diet is only one piece of the bigger puzzle. It will only be optimally effective when you implement it in combination with all the other principles and recommendations in this book.

Rationale for the GFCF Diet

The GFCF diet has been controversial, but I'll tell you why it's a great first step in significantly improving your child's wellbeing.

First, I'll address the fact that the scientific evidence does not yet *fully* support the GFCF diet's efficacy. Then, I'll discuss the many reasons why it should *still* be the foundation diet, at least during the initial stages of your child's health-building program.

Why Research on GFCF Diets in ASD is Inconclusive

While a subset of autistic children definitely benefit from GFCF diets, scientific data remains inconclusive as to the diet's effectiveness.[2][3] Some potential reasons why this is the case include:

- Studies often look for improvement in "autistic symptoms". That's not what we're after at all. We want to improve your child's health - that is our goal. Furthermore, many of the studies are too short. For example, a 12-week trial may find no significant evidence of improvement, but that should be the MINIMUM trial period before you would expect to see results. Six months is probably better. Concluding that the diet is ineffective from an 8- or 12-week trial is short-sighted. (Unfortunately, it's usually the people interpreting the study results, rather than the researchers, that come to these conclusions.)
- It is unclear how well the parents stuck to the diets in the studies. If they didn't follow through well, it can easily skew the researchers' results negatively.
- A lot of gluten-free substitutes such as corn, soy, or legumes may cause reactions which detract from the benefits of the GFCF diet.
- If the children in the studies had other underlying health problems (e.g. gut infections, leaky gut, other food sensitivities), then it is less likely that changing a couple of variables in the diet would have a significant positive effect. A more holistic approach is necessary in the real world, though it does not lend itself to scientific research very well.

Let me expand on the first point above. Just because an "intervention" does not reduce autistic symptoms on paper (in a study), does that mean we should dismiss it?

Here's how it works: researchers hypothesise that an intervention (e.g. GFCF diet, or supplementing certain vitamins, minerals, or essential fatty acids) may be a good "treatment" for autism and devise an experiment to try it out. They look at how effective said treatment is at lowering symptoms on an ASD rating scale such as CARS or other methodology used to diagnose and assess autism.

If the outcome of the study finds that the intervention does not lower ASD symptoms significantly, the authors of the paper will state that in the paper. People that read the paper may conclude that the intervention is not worthwhile.

But is that really smart? What if the children's overall health improved in the study? What if a metabolic imbalance was corrected? What if the microbiota and immune system became more resilient? Those subtle details are often missed or omitted because the researchers have a specific goal they are working towards and they use fairly rigid means to assess the effectiveness of the intervention being studied (e.g. checklists, rating scales).

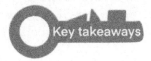

Key takeaways

My point here is that we should not automatically dismiss something on the basis that "the evidence does not fully support it", because the research generally looks at "does it lower autism symptoms?" It might not, but it may have many other health benefits!

Once again, my intent with this book is to help you get your child as healthy as possible. We use diet and supplements to help us achieve that goal. If some symptoms do improve as a result of better health, then we can consider that a welcome bonus.

Having said that, I will present any relevant evidence (where available) because I believe it will support the recommendations in the book and will expand your knowledge on the topics we discuss.

Potential Benefits of the GFCF Diet

There are several potential benefits to the gluten-free, casein-free (and soy-free) diet. We'll cover some of these topics in more depth in this section, but in a nutshell, the rationale is:

- Many children have sensitivities to gluten and casein (this causes inflammation in the gut and immune reactions). These may not show up on basic food sensitivities tests due to reasons we discussed in the previous chapter.
- Antibodies to gluten and cow's milk proteins have the potential

to cross-react with our body's tissues, which can cause tissue damage, inflammation, and autoimmune reactions.

- Opiate-like peptides (similar to morphine) can form during incomplete digestion of gluten and casein. These can exert negative effects on behaviour and health by binding to opiate receptors in the brain.
- Soy is often genetically modified, inflammatory, sprayed with chemicals, and can mimic certain negative effects of gluten and casein. It is best to exclude it from the diet also, at least for the trial period to ensure benefits are not negated.
- The GFCF diet can help to normalise a leaky gut.[4]
- An added benefit of the GFCF is you avoid some mycotoxins that often contaminate cereal and milk products.[5]

Where the Science Does Support the GFCF Diet

Various studies of the GFCF diet in ASD over the years have observed improvements in the following areas:[6]

- Communication and use of language
- Attention and concentration
- Social integration and interaction
- Self-injurious behaviour or altered pain perception
- Repetitive or stereotyped patterns of behaviour
- Motor co-ordination
- Hyperactivity

When it comes to research on the diet, longer studies (e.g. 12 months) seem to show positive results more so than shorter trials (e.g. 12 weeks).

For example, a two-stage, randomised, controlled study with autistic children reported significant improvements in core autistic and related behaviours after 8 and 12 months on a GFCF diet.[3] The benefits reported were in communication sub-scores on the ADOS evaluation, while the parents noticed improvements in social interaction, daily living skills, inattention, and hyperactivity.

One survey of 387 parents of autistic children who had tried the GFCF diet reported that those families who were stricter in implementing the diet had better results. Hardly surprising. The children showed greater improvement in autistic behaviours, physiological symptoms, and social behaviours. The researchers also reported that the diet was more effective at improving these factors when the children had GI symptoms, food allergy diagnoses, or suspected food sensitivities to begin with.[7]

This research indicates that kids with gastrointestinal problems may be more likely to benefit from GFCF diets.

Another study found that autistic individuals on wheat and dairy-free diets had significantly lower intestinal permeability than those not on such diets.[8]

Parent Reported Benefits

Research is helpful to have when making significant decisions about your child's diet, but we don't always need scientific evidence to know something is beneficial. Do you need a study to tell you that touching a hot stove will hurt? You can read all the studies in the world that report the health benefits of broccoli, but if you feel horrible after eating it, would you force yourself to continue eating it? Surely, not just because the "science supports it".

Many families have had great success with the GFCF and have decided to use it long term. That's what we call being "evidence-based, but not evidence-limited". We can examine the scientific literature but don't have to automatically dismiss everything that is not yet fully supported by it.

If we had to wait for all the science to be done and 100% conclusive, we would be waiting for a long time. Then, don't forget, we need to wait for the clinicians to begin applying it (which can take decades).

Parent-reported benefits of the GFCF diet include:

- Improved gastrointestinal function (less constipation and diarrhoea)
- Better sleep
- Less irritability, hyperactivity, and stimulatory behaviours
- Decreased emotional volatility and improved mood
- Increased appetite for other foods
- Fewer rashes or skin issues
- Less runny noses and other allergic-type reactions
- Improved verbalisation, eye contact, and attention

At this point, we have scientific data and anecdotal evidence supporting the notion that a GFCF diet should at least be given a try for a reasonable period of time (at least 3 to 6 months). If you see no benefits from going GFCF, simply re-introduce the foods previously excluded, knowing you gave it a good attempt.

However, as you'll see shortly, by going through the exercise of implementing the GFCF diet, you won't just be excluding gluten and casein - you will be improving many other aspects of your child's nutrition. So, while you may eventually decide to bring back wheat or milk products, you will find that your child's new baseline diet has improved considerably.

Potential Problems with Gluten and Grains

Gluten is a group of proteins found in wheat, barley, rye, and triticale. It is a collective name we use for proteins such as various gliadins and glutenins, about 70 of them in total.

So, what's the problem with gluten? Apart from it being one of the most common food allergens, gluten is difficult for humans to digest, especially if our microbiota or gut lining are compromised. In fact, all grains, if not processed properly, can be problematic. I've summarised the main points below.

Potential problems with gluten:[4][9-14]

- There are many components of gluten to which your child can react, however, most basic food sensitivities tests don't test for them.
- Your child may not present with gastrointestinal symptoms if they react to gluten, making it difficult to identify a sensitivity.
- Incomplete digestion of gluten can cause the formation of opioid-like peptides (gluteomorphins). They can travel through the blood to your child's brain and cause changes in behaviour.
- Parts of gluten can mimic the structure of some of our body's tissues, including those in the brain. This can cause immune activation that can lead to tissue damage, inflammation, and autoimmunity. (We touched on this in Chapter Two)
- A leaky gut can make all the above much worse. Gluten can also contribute to leaky gut, thus instigating a vicious cycle.

As you can see, problems can manifest in many ways and your child won't necessarily have gut distress if they are intolerant to the various proteins found in gluten.

Further issues with grains exist, such as:

- Today's wheat is highly hybridised and contains more gluten.
- There are many other non-gluten proteins and lectins in grains that may cause immune reactions in your child.
- As discussed in Chapter Five, non-organic grains are heavily sprayed with herbicides, pesticides, artificial fertilisers, and other chemicals that contribute to your child's toxic load.
- Grains that have not been prepared properly by soaking, sprouting, or fermentation contain anti-nutrients including trypsin inhibitors, tannins, and phytate. These can inhibit digestive enzymes in the gut and impair digestion, or can bind with minerals such as zinc, iron, and magnesium and inhibit their absorption.

Hopefully, you're starting to see why removing gluten from the diet, at least while your child's gut health is improving, is so crucial.

Potential Problems with Dairy

Milk proteins such as casein are problematic for a significant subset of autistic children.[4][9][15] Casein can contribute to gut inflammation and immune reactivity. It may also bind with human tissues or cause cross-reactions due to molecular mimicry.[16]

Apart from casein, other milk protein constituents that have been shown to cause immune responses in autistic children include α-lactalbumin and β-lactoglobulin.[17] On top of that, some kids may be intolerant to lactose, the sugar in milk.

In addition, conventional dairy has the following problems:

- If not organic or pastured, chances are high that the animals are fed grains (which may be genetically modified and sprayed with herbicides and pesticides), hormones, antibiotics, and other chemicals that are likely to contaminate the final product to an extent.
- Pasteurisation can make the calcium in dairy less bioavailable and reduce the nutritional value.
- Synthetic vitamins are often added to milk products to increase the perceived nutrient content. However, these are never going to be as good for your child as whole-food sources of those vitamins.

Opioid Peptides

Opioid peptides are morphine-like compounds that are formed when gluten and casein are not properly digested. (A peptide is simply a chain of amino acids, the building block of proteins). When peptides originate outside the body, we call them exorphins, or exogenous opioids. When they are produced in the body, we call them endorphins. You may have heard that our bodies can produce endorphins that make us feel good (such as when we exercise).

Gluteomorphins and casomorphins can be formed due to digestive enzyme insufficiencies or an otherwise compromised gut lining. They can enter the bloodstream and make their way to your child's brain, where the effects tend not to be desirable. Opioids can exert strong behavioural effects and are often found in high levels in the urine or blood of autistic children.[18-28]

Some effects exerted by opioid peptides can include:[5][9][29-37]

- Increasing ASD symptoms
- Increases in aggression, self-abusive behaviour, lack of attention, or sleepiness
- Increased inflammation in the gut
- Lower antioxidant levels (e.g. glutathione)
- Contributing to oxidative stress
- Exerting a negative influence on the gastrointestinal, immune, and nervous systems
- Interfering with methylation and DNA expression
- Affecting certain neurotransmitter systems (with potential behavioural effects)

Whether opioid peptides become a problem for your child depends on many factors, such as:[29]

- Genetic predisposition
- Early life exposure to environmental toxins and other stressors
- State of their gut's health and level of intestinal permeability
- Digestive enzyme activity in the gut
- Increased blood-brain barrier permeability

When excessive opioids are indeed an issue, GFCF diets have been shown to provide significant improvement in autistic children.[25][38-40]

Potential Risks of GFCF Diets

After covering the negative aspects of gluten and conventional dairy, you might not be surprised to hear that there aren't many downsides to the GFCF diet, apart from the logistical difficulty of implementing it in the real world.

Let's briefly discuss the most common nutritional risks with going gluten and casein-free, as well as how you can address them.

Lack of Dietary Calcium

One of the few drawbacks of the GFCF diet is that removing dairy products from your child's diet can greatly reduce their calcium intake. As you know, calcium is crucial for building strong bones, but it also plays many other vital roles in the body.

As we discussed earlier in the book, adequate calcium intake and status is also important to prevent lead toxicity,[41][42] so you'll need to make sure you supplement your child regularly. I'll explain how to do that in Chapter Ten.

Nutrients Used to Fortify Wheat Flour

Refined wheat flour has been fortified with micronutrients to prevent deficiencies for many decades now. These usually include iron, zinc, folic acid, and other B vitamins.

When you take out fortified wheat from the diet, you need to make sure that *if* it was the source of those nutrients, they are added back into the diet via other sources.

But we will take it a step further with the *Autism Wellbeing Plan*. Not only will you improve your child's diet to the point where you won't have to rely on fortified nutrients, you will also supplement them with more bioavailable forms of vitamins and minerals than the cheap stuff they put in our food (and pretend makes up for the deficits). A two-fold improvement.

For example, flour is often fortified with folic acid, cyanocobalamin (vitamin B_{12}), and zinc oxide. These are the lowest quality forms of these nutrients you can find. As you will see in later chapters, the vitamins and minerals you'll use will be of much higher quality and bioavailability.

Lack of Dietary Fibre

It's important to keep your child pooping regularly to avoid accumulation and absorption of toxic metabolites in their gut. Grain products do provide some fibre, which helps to feed the beneficial gut bacteria and move the stool along the digestive tract.

As you take out gluten-containing grains (or potentially all grains, if you're on a more advanced diet), it's crucial to plan for adding some fibre back into your child's diet.

Luckily, it's not difficult. All you need to do is ensure your child gets a steady stream of whole fruits and vegetables. You may also want to add in a prebiotic fibre such as inulin at a certain point, but please discuss this with your practitioner as the state of the gut and microbiota needs to be considered carefully before adding prebiotics to the diet.

Implementing the Healthy GFCF

The initial stages of introducing the GFCF diet may be quite challenging for you if wheat and dairy products are a staple for your child. You need to be prepared.

Your child may experience some withdrawal symptoms for days, or even weeks. But that should make you think, are foods that cause such symptoms so good to begin with? You don't get withdrawal symptoms quitting apples or lamb chops.

On top of that, you may encounter some tantrums, pleading, or crying along the way. But you need to stay strong knowing why you're doing all this. Remember that this is only a temporary measure. The quicker and stricter you are with your child's health-building program, the quicker they will get healthier and you can start to loosen up some of the stringent restrictions.

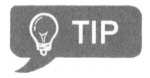

To minimise the stress for you and your child, it's best to introduce the GFCF diet gradually, especially if they like a lot of dairy or gluten-containing foods.

With older children, you can sit down with them and explain what you are trying to accomplish with these dietary changes. Explain to them the health benefits that are possible by following the diet. Make them feel included. A proactive participant in this journey.

If you're worried about the social aspect of it, such as "Is my child going to fit in with their friends or school-mates?", please remember that we live in a time where so many people are doing the gluten-free lifestyle, that there is no longer a stigma attached to it. Families everywhere are excluding certain foods from their children's diets due to personal preferences, food allergies, or sensitivities.

Steps to Take

Use the following guidelines when implementing the GFCF diet:

- Begin by removing dairy products (except grass-fed butter).
- Do it gradually and allow one to three weeks for your child to get accustomed.
- Start swapping in gluten-free products for breads, cereals, snacks and other foods your child eats until you have replaced all gluten-containing products.
- Remove soy-based products as soon as feasible for your family (if you use a lot of soy-based foods, you may want to reduce them gradually, otherwise just stop buying them).
- Phase out the gluten-free substitutes for healthier foods.

Once you've done the above steps, you would then continue to refine, improve, and diversify the diet by gradually reducing sugary, processed, and junk foods, and replacing them with healthier whole-food alternatives.

Depending on your time, energy, and motivation, it can take from two to eight weeks to implement the diet fully. It also depends on how quickly you can wean your child off the wheat and dairy-based foods - it's easier with some kids than others.

The refining process you can take your time with, as long as you stick to organic foods. Organic snacks are a lot less detrimental than the non-organic garbage that fills our grocery stores.

Foods to Avoid

The foods we'll cover in this section pertain specifically to the healthy

GFCF diet. In the next chapter, I'll go into more depth on how to clean up your child's diet to reduce exposure to harmful chemicals as much as possible.

The key foods to avoid are:

- **Grains:** barley, bulgur, corn, couscous, rye, oats, soy, spelt, wheat, bran, durum, semolina, and all products derived from them
- **Dairy:** everything except grass-fed butter
- **Snacks:** biscuits, crackers, ice-cream, granola bars, cakes, and other sweets and packaged foods
- **Staples:** bread and breaded foods, cereals, and pastas

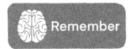

Remember that corn and soy are best to be avoided during the initial trial of the diet to prevent potential cross reactions. In any case, if you ever decide to feed your child corn or soy products, they must always be organically grown to avoid GMOs and harmful chemicals.

Of course, if you have tested your child for food sensitivities, you would also need to exclude the moderate and highly reactive foods from their diet.

Hidden Sources of Gluten

Gluten is commonly used as a food additive or thickener. Products that often contain it include:

- Processed foods
- Baked beans
- Ice cream
- Soy sauce
- Syrups and gravies
- Dressings including ketchup, mayonnaise, and malt vinegar
- Ready-made soups

- Deli meat
- Veggie burgers and imitation meats

You will want to seek out products that are specifically labelled as gluten-free, because it is often hidden under non-obvious names, such as:

- Hydrolysed vegetable protein
- Modified food starch
- Soy protein
- Maltodextrin
- Brown rice syrup
- Triticum vulgare or aestivum
- Natural flavouring
- Hydrolysate
- Hydrolysed malt extract
- Yeast extract

Any time you see the above ingredients on a label, try to think about why you are considering purchasing that item, and whether a healthier whole-food option is available nearby.

Hidden Sources of Casein

Keep an eye out for calcium caseinate, potassium caseinate, and sodium caseinate (also called casein sodium, sodium complexes, casein sodium salt), which are common additives in many processed foods, such as:

- Baked goods
- Ice cream, doughnuts, chocolate, and other deserts
- Ham, sausages, fish cakes, and other meat products

Food Substitutions

Most fruits and vegetables, as well as all animal products except dairy, are allowed on the GFCF diet. Smart substitutions you can make include:

- Gluten-free grains such as amaranth, millet, rice, quinoa, teff, or sorghum instead of wheat
- Organic coconut or rice milk instead of cow's milk
- Sea salt instead of table salt

- Stevia, xylitol, or honey instead of sugar
- Butter from grass-fed cows instead of margarine or other vegetable spreads
- Medium-chain triglycerides (MCT) oil, organic coconut oil, and organic extra virgin olive oil instead of vegetable and seed oils
- You can use fruits, nuts, and homemade healthy ice-creams and desserts for snacks

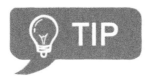

As you implement the diet, try not to become overly reliant on processed foods or gluten-free alternatives that may still contain a lot of sugar and other undesirable ingredients. Cooking meals yourself from scratch is the best way to control what ingredients make it onto your child's plate.

Common Pitfalls in Implementing the Diet

A well-planned GFCF diet is not too complicated in theory but may prove to be more challenging in practice due to many factors including:

- Your child's temperament and food preferences
- Your own energy and willpower to continue doing the diet
- External influences may inadvertently sabotage your progress (friends, family, schools, corporations marketing junk food to kids)

Below are the most common mistakes families make when implementing the GFCF diet:

- Expecting results too soon (give it at least 3 to 6 months)
- Using gluten-free products as permanent staples
- Using products with too much sugar
- Continuing to use a lot of processed or junk foods
- Eating foods contaminated with gluten (or with hidden sources

of gluten)
- Not enough variety in the diet
- Not sticking to the diet strictly

If you do not seem to notice any benefits from the diet in terms of your child's health, think about the above points and whether there may be some improvements you can make. Also consider other variables such as food sensitivities or unaddressed gut infections that may be hindering your child's progress.

Expanding the Diet

It's up to you and your practitioner to decide when to begin expanding your child's diet. Unfortunately, some families see little benefit by going GFCF, and are anxious to get back to normalcy. Others decide to continue with it indefinitely because it is so beneficial for their child. In many cases, because the parents go on the GFCF diet themselves to support their child, everyone in the family feels much better.

First off, you should not start re-introducing gluten or casein if your child still has:

- Noticeable gut dysfunction (constipation, diarrhoea, gas, bloating)
- Gut dysbiosis or you are doing a pathogen eradication protocol
- Leaky gut, elevated antibodies to gut barrier proteins, or sensitivities to gluten or casein evidenced by lab testing

If your child's health has improved considerably after three to six months on the diet, you may decide to try some foods that contain gluten or casein to see if you notice a reaction or behavioural changes. Or, more likely, you may find yourself in a situation where cheat foods are readily available, such as a birthday party or other celebration.

The most important thing to keep in mind is that reactions will often not be immediate. So, keep a close eye on your child over the next couple of days and note any changes in behaviour, mood, sleep, or other clues that they may be having a delayed reaction.

It may also be the case that a small amount of dairy or gluten doesn't affect your child noticeably in the short term, and it's only after resuming regular intake of those foods that their health starts deteriorating. You need to remain vigilant, which is why it's useful to keep a journal where you can track diet, supplements, and subtle changes over time. (I'll remind you about this in Chapter Twelve.)

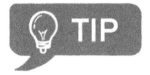

Running a food sensitivities panel several months after re-introducing wheat and dairy is usually a good idea because you won't necessarily notice if your child is experiencing inflammation and immune reactivity.

More Advanced Diets

It may be warranted to graduate your child to a more advanced diet in some cases. The decision will be based on your child's unique case, lab test results, and your practitioner's recommendations.

In this section, I'll give you a brief overview of several diets used in ASD. Each has its place and appropriate usage. Some are only meant to be used short or mid-term to correct an imbalance, while others may need to be followed long-term.

You will find further information and links to resources on the diets discussed on the resources webpage for this book.

Low Oxalate Diet

I cover what oxalates are in Chapter Four, how to test for them in Chapter Six, and some supplements that can help to address them in Chapter Eleven.

When the oxalate markers are elevated on the organic acids test, it most often calls for a low oxalate diet (LOD) to be implemented.

The LOD reduces the oxalate content of your child's diet slowly (5-10% per week) over the course of several weeks or months. You would need to analyse what high oxalate foods your child eats and gradually reduce them. It's important to take your time with this because a sudden reduction can result in the body dumping oxalates out of its tissues, which can be an uncomfortable or even painful process.

Examples of the foods with the highest oxalate content include almonds, amaranth, beets, buckwheat, carrots, chard, chia seeds, chocolate, cocoa, nuts, parsnips, potatoes, sweet potatoes, rhubarb, sesame seeds, soy, spinach, spelt, and wheat. (Yes, a lot of staples in our modern diet can be problematic for many autistic kids.)

The LOD follows this basic process:

- Learn which foods are high in oxalate
- Use diet logs to determine which of those foods are in your child's diet (I'll show you a simple way to track your child's diet in Chapter Twelve)
- Begin to reduce oxalate-containing foods by 5-10% per week
- In most cases, you would use some supplements outlined in Chapter Eleven and an anti-fungal protocol, if a test indicates yeast or mould are an issue for your child (certain fungal species can produce oxalate crystals)
- Once your child's gut has healed and overall health is improved, you may slowly introduce some previously excluded foods (but you'll likely need to keep the oxalate content in their diet lower than before)

Specific Carbohydrate Diet

The Specific Carbohydrate Diet (SCD) diet is often used when celiac disease or inflammatory bowel disease (IBD) are present (such as Crohn's disease or ulcerative colitis). It can also help in chronic diarrhoea cases.

The SCD diet restricts all grains and complex carbohydrates (starches), as well as two-sugar molecules such as table sugar. The only sugars it allows are monosaccharides (glucose, fructose, galactose) from fruits, honey, and non-starchy vegetables.

The diet centres around meat, eggs, natural cheeses, nuts, fruits, some legumes, and certain vegetables (e.g. onions, spinach, peppers, cauliflower, and cabbage).

GAPS Diet

The GAPS (Gut and Psychology Syndrome) diet is similar to the Specific Carbohydrate Diet, though it is slightly more restrictive and systematic in terms of its implementation.

Dr Natasha Campbell-McBride introduced the diet with her book "Gut and Psychology Syndrome: Natural Treatment for Autism, Dyspraxia, A.D.D., Dyslexia, A.D.H.D., Depression, Schizophrenia". Many families have had great success with the diet since Dr Campbell-McBride published her book.

The GAPS diet restricts all grains, commercial dairy, starchy vegetables, and all processed or refined carbohydrates. The diet consists of mainly meats, fish, eggs, fermented foods, and vegetables.

Low FODMAP Diet

FODMAP stands for "fermentable oligo-, di-, mono-saccharides and polyols". They are short chain carbohydrates that are resistant to digestion in the small intestine, so we rely on our gut bacteria to ferment them. FODMAPs also draw a lot of water into them, which can affect intestinal motility, stool formation, and bowel movement frequency.

People can become sensitive to FODMAPs, which can cause digestive symptoms such as gas, bloating, stomach pain, diarrhoea, or constipation. That's when a low FODMAP diet may be in order.

Many foods contain FODMAPs, so implementing a low FODMAP diet takes considerable research and planning. Example of FODMAPs include:

- Fructose (found in fruits and table sugar)
- Lactose (the sugar in milk)
- Sugar alcohols such as sorbitol, mannitol, xylitol, and maltitol
- Fructans and galactans, found in some grains or legumes

Low FODMAP foods include meat, eggs, rice, and certain fruits, vegetables, and nuts. A more complete list is available on the book's resources webpage.

FAILSAFE Diet

FAILSAFE stands for Free of Additives, Low in Salicylates, Amines and Flavour Enhancers. The diet was originally designed for ADHD, but people with other conditions have benefited by implementing it.

The FAILSAFE diet is rather strict. It restricts most processed foods and additives such as colours, flavours, preservatives, and antioxidants, as well as many other chemicals such as salicylates and amines that are found in various foods.

Salicylates are compounds in plants that protect them from predators and disease. They can also be found in medications, perfumes, and preservatives. Some people are more sensitive to salicylates and feel considerable improvement in many symptoms after eliminating them from their diet and environment.

Foods allowed on the FAILSAFE diet include fresh meats (not vacuum-packed or aged), dairy and some grains (if tolerated), and specific fruits and vegetables.

Feingold Diet

The Feingold diet is less strict than the FAILSAFE diet. It eliminates some foods that contain salicylates, phenols, and other additives. Phenols may contribute to aggression, hyperactivity, impulsivity, sleep issues, or self-injurious behaviour. When removed from the diet, parents often see improvements in their children.

Examples of foods or additives restricted on the Feingold diet include:

- Salicylates: almonds, apples, cucumbers, honey, peppers, pineapple, plums, tomatoes.
- Phenols: food additives such as BHA, BHT, other preservatives, artificial colours or flavours, MSG, nitrates, nitrites, and corn syrup.

Ketogenic Diet

The ketogenic diet is a high-fat, low-carbohydrate, and low-to-moderate protein diet. It was originally developed to help control seizures in epilepsy, but evidence is emerging that it can be used with benefit in some neurological conditions, including ASD.[43-45]

On a high-fat ketogenic diet, the body is forced to start burning fat for fuel because the dietary carbohydrates are not enough to meet its needs. The body starts making ketone bodies, which it can use as an energy source instead of glucose.

The ketogenic diet has its place in the right circumstances, but it can be challenging to follow in practice. It must always be implemented under the care of an experienced clinician.

Wrap-up

After spending the previous six chapters looking at the myriad of ways your child's health can be challenged and ways of identifying them, we finally get to the "doing" part of the *Autism Wellbeing Plan*.

In this chapter, you learnt about the potential benefits the GFCF diet can bring your child, and its role in their health-building program. I gave you a simple framework for implementing the diet and some tips to help ensure your success with it. Finally, we took a brief tour of more advanced diets, and situations in which you may utilise them.

As I mentioned before, the GFCF is just one piece of the puzzle. There are many "versions" of it, some healthy and others not-so-unhealthy. You certainly want to stay on the healthy side as much as possible.

But it's not always that simple. You also need to learn to protect your child from the myriad of toxic exposures in our modern environment and food supply. We'll discuss how to do that in the next chapter.

CHAPTER EIGHT: CLEANING UP YOUR CHILD'S DIET AND ENVIRONMENT

Overview of this Chapter

In this chapter, I'll offer some strategies you can use to clean up your child's diet and environment from the countless toxic substances to which they are exposed.

By reading this book, my intent is to bring you through the various stages of learning new (and potentially shocking) information.

If much of what we discussed in Chapter Five was new to you, I don't want you to linger in any state of shock, fear, disappointment, anger, or helplessness for too long. Sure, we all may go through these stages when learning about what our world has become (or rather, what big corporations have done to it in the name of profit). But I want to inform you so that you may become empowered, and hopefully, optimistic about the future.

I say this because too many people get stuck in one of two dualities when confronted with the reality of our toxic environment. Some are completely paralysed into inaction due to fear, denial, or continued ignorance of the dangers. Others go the other extreme of trying to reduce all toxic exposures - an impossible task in today's world and a sure-fire way to alienate yourself from your friends and loved ones.

We want to strike a happy medium where you can reduce the major sources of harmful exposure to your child and family, but don't have to throw out or replace everything you own (or relocate to a remote mountain village).

Having said that, there are no two ways about it - the task of cleaning up your child's diet and environment will be a significant challenge. It will require lifestyle and habit changes, which may be harder for you than your child.

But on the upside, they will be positive changes in the long term, so it's worth getting excited about this process.

It does get easier, I promise you.

Principles of Cleaning Up the Diet and Environment

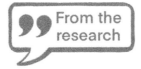

"Toxicants implicated in ASD included pesticides, phthalates, polychlorinated biphenyls (PCBs), solvents, toxic waste sites, air pollutants and heavy metals, with the strongest evidence found for air pollutants and pesticides."[1]

The principles of cleaning up your child's diet and environment are simple, though they are not always easy in practice.

The common themes throughout this chapter are:

- Eat organic whole foods
- Cook as many meals from scratch as possible
- Avoid processed foods
- Avoid plastics as much as possible
- Replace conventional cleaning products, soaps, shampoos, and other products with safer alternatives that are free from harsh chemicals

Using the Environmental Working Group's Resources

Before we get into the practical aspects of reducing your family's toxic exposure, I would urge you to get acquainted with the Environmental Working Group's website, where you will find much more in-depth information on the topic. They have a rich bank of consumer guides on how to shop for food and products such as cleaning supplies, water filters, and sunscreen.

One of their most valuable resources is the Food Scores database of over 80,000 products, rated on nutrition, ingredients, and processing. You can search for foods your family consumes regularly to see how they stack up. Foods are scored from 1 to 10, with 10 being the worst rating.

For example, if a product has ingredients that may be from genetically modified crops and questionable additives such as preservatives, its score is likely to be closer to 10, which means you're best off avoiding it.

Summary of Reasons to Eat ONLY Organic Food

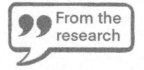
From the research

"In conclusion, we were able to demonstrate that an organic diet provides a dramatic and immediate protective effect against exposures to organophosphorus pesticides that are commonly used in agricultural production."[2]

Please do not underestimate the value of an organic diet and the potential dangers of conventionally grown industrial food. Organic foods are grown and processed without the use of artificial fertilisers, pesticides, herbicides (like glyphosate), hormones, and antibiotics. By going organic you will dramatically decrease your child's exposure to these, and other harmful chemicals and additives.[2][3]

By way of logic and evidence, I hope I can convince you that an all-organic diet should be the foundation of your child's health-building program. It is a non-negotiable, foundational intervention, especially in the United States, where the use of toxic chemicals in agriculture has reached insane levels.

Here is the simple, but convincing, three-point case for an all-organic diet:

1. Herbicides and pesticides are harmful to humans (links with autism, neurodevelopmental problems, cancer, and other disorders).
2. Conventionally produced industrial food is heavily sprayed with herbicides and pesticides.
3. Therefore, organic food is the *only* safe choice, given the evidence we're presented.

The problem (and beauty) of information is that once you know something, you can't unknow it. I will never look at a conventionally farmed piece of meat and not feel an aversion to it. Likewise, a fruit or vegetable. Just knowing that I have no idea what the farmers were feeding the animal, or spraying the produce with, creates an unease that cannot be reconciled with how good a product looks.

I hope that you, too, will learn to look at food through a similar lens. When you go to the grocery store, you are making one of two choices. On one hand, you can make every plateful of food nourishing and supportive for your child. On the other, it could be a plate loaded with toxins that put a burden on their health.

Even something as innocent-looking as a juice-box or breakfast cereal could have significant levels of pesticides and herbicides in it. Always remember that the mass-produced industrial quantities of juices and snacks are so cheap due to many sacrifices in quality and cutting of corners. Unfortunately, you and your family will pay the price for these profit-enhancing measures, unless you make changes in your buying habits.

Let's summarise the major reasons supporting an organic diet for your child, before moving on to the rest of the topics in this chapter:

- **Reduction of herbicides and pesticides.** Organic foods have considerably lower levels of herbicides, pesticides, fungicides, and other potentially harmful chemicals. As you saw in Chapter Five, a multitude of chemicals implicated in ASD and other conditions are sprayed on crops with reckless abandon.
- **Avoidance of genetically modified (GM) foods** such as soy, corn, canola, sugar beets, and others.
- **Avoidance of hormones and antibiotics.** Pastured animals are much healthier than their feedlot counterparts. An animal that eats grass will usually have a better omega-3 to omega-6 fatty acid profile (omega-3s are more anti-inflammatory while omega-6s fatty acids tend to be more pro-inflammatory). The feed used for organically raised livestock is grown without the use of synthetic fertilisers or pesticides, and GM crops are never used. The animals are allowed to roam free outside in the fresh air and sunshine, and are not given antibiotics or growth hormones.
- **Reducing heavy metal exposure.** Certain heavy metals (such as mercury and arsenic) are very effective anti-microbial and anti-fungal agents. Thus, they are often added to products used in conventional agriculture to slow down the growth of fungi and bacteria. For example, mercury is added to the feed used in fish farming and is sometimes added to seeds to preserve them.
- **Potentially more nutritional than conventional food.**

This last point may not sit well with you. Doesn't organic food have similar nutrition to non-organic food? Isn't it only the pesticides and other chemicals that we're avoiding? I fear that we may have been victims of the conventional agriculture industry's propaganda on that one.

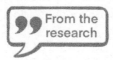
From the research

"In conclusion, organic crops, on average, have higher concentrations of antioxidants, lower concentrations of Cd and a lower incidence of pesticide residues than the non-organic comparators across regions and production seasons."[4]

The above quote is from an extensive meta-analysis based on 343 peer-reviewed publications that showed meaningful differences in the composition of organic and non-organic foods. That's not one or two studies, it's hundreds of them!

The researchers concluded that not only does organic food have less pesticide residues and cadmium, it tends to have higher levels of antioxidants. In the paper, they state:

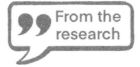

From the research

"Based on the differences reported, results indicate that a switch from conventional to organic crop consumption would result in a 20-40 % (and for some compounds more than 60 %) increase in crop-based antioxidant/(poly)phenolic intake levels without a simultaneous increase in energy, which would be in line with the dietary recommendations"[4]

Wouldn't it be great to eat the same quantity of food, but receive 20% to 40% (or even 60%) more antioxidants from it? Sign me up. The benefit for kids is that they eat little food in terms of volume, so the more nutrition you can cram into every bite, the better.

But do you know what? Just avoiding all the chemicals in non-organic food is more than ample motive to switch to an all-organic diet. Any benefits above and beyond that we can consider a welcome bonus.

Let's conclude this discussion on the merits of an organic diet and the dangers of conventional foods. Hopefully, you've come to the realisation that organic products are worth the extra cost, and the money saved on cheaper non-organic foods is a false economy that will come back to bite you.

Transitioning to an Organic Diet

Let's face it, not all families can make the immediate switch to an all-organic diet, either due to cost or logistical issues. While it's the best choice for your child (and you) to do it as quickly as possible, I'll outline some strategies to help you make a gradual transition.

The important first step is to remove the foods that are most likely to be sources of toxic exposure. Once you have those basics under control, you can start swapping in other organic products.

Animal Foods

As you make the transition to only pasture-raised and wild-caught animal foods, keep the following points in mind:

- **Organic or pastured eggs** are an amazing food, packed full of nutrients and well worth the extra cost. This is perhaps the quickest substitution you can make, if your child tolerates them. Remember not to overcook the yolk, as it oxidises the fats, which is not desirable. The best way to prepare eggs is with runny yolks.
- **No farmed fish.** Please do your family a favour and never buy farmed fish, including organic farmed salmon. Small wild-caught fish like sardines are inexpensive and are an infinitely better option. You can get them fresh or canned, and they can be eaten 3-4 times a week as a source of protein and omega-3 fatty acids.
- **Organically raised ground beef** is cheaper than steaks and is a versatile food to make meatballs, burgers, and stews or stir-frys.
- **Chicken giblets such as necks, liver, and hearts** are usually cheap to buy organic, and are suitable for soups or to separate into small portions and freeze. You can then cook small amounts to add a nutrient boost to meals. Liver from younger animals (like chicken) is preferable than older ones, such as cows. Please note that liver is high in copper, and high copper is common in autistic children. If you don't know your child's copper status, or you know it's high, don't overdo it with the liver (twice a week is more than enough) until you have balanced the zinc-to-copper ratio.
- **Organic chicken wings, thighs, and giblets** are cheaper than whole chickens or breast. Use them in soups or simply grill them, and the kids can eat them with their hands. The great part about organic chicken wings and thighs is all that skin is packed full of collagen and glycine, which are great for the gut, joints, skin, and have many other benefits in the body.

- **Many stores discount meats as they approach their sell-by date**, often within a day or two. This is a great way to get higher-quality organic meat at lower prices. If you buy a few packets, you can freeze and use them later.

Plant Foods

If you're entirely new to eating organic and are only beginning to make the transition, I'd highly recommend you check out the Environmental Working Group's (EWG) Clean Fifteen and Dirty Dozen lists.

The Clean Fifteen is a list of the least-sprayed fruits and vegetables, while the Dirty Dozen are the most sprayed. You want to ensure you never buy the Dirty Dozen, unless they've been grown organically. You may opt for the foods on the Clean Fifteen until you've made the full transition to an all-organic diet.

The lists apply to the US, but you can still use them as a guide if you live elsewhere. Farming practises are not all that different around the world nowadays. The EWG update their lists yearly. To give you a quick preview, below are some foods from both lists from 2019.

EWG's Clean Fifteen:

- Avocadoes
- Onions
- Asparagus
- Cabbage
- Mushrooms
- Broccoli
- Cauliflower
- Kiwis

Some of the EWG's Dirty Dozen foods (always buy organic):

- Spinach
- Strawberries
- Grapes
- Apples
- Peaches
- Pears
- Tomatoes
- Potatoes
- Nectarines

Do you notice anything striking about the foods I've listed from the Dirty Dozen? That's right, the most sprayed foods are also some of the foods we eat the most!

Avoid Unfiltered Tap Water at All Costs

When it comes to water, spring water is your best choice. If you cannot find spring water in your area (including bottled in your local supermarkets, which is still better than tap water, even if in plastic bottles), then carbon-filtered tap water is your next viable option.

Although a Brita jug won't filter out all the contaminants in your tap water, it certainly is better than doing nothing at all. The best thing to do is invest in a high-quality water filtration system for your home, if at all possible. Until then, you may want to consider a filter that attaches to your faucet, so you can run your tap water through it and a carbon-filter jug for extra precaution. Faucet attachments are inexpensive and can reduce many harmful compounds including chlorine, fluoride, lead, arsenic, PCBs, and other common pollutants.

Don't Forget the Bathroom

How bad is the water in your bathroom, really? Well, you wouldn't drink it, would you?

Remember that chlorine and other contaminants are volatile, which means they can evaporate from the water into the surrounding air while you're bathing your child. They can inhale them and absorb them through the skin.

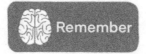

You may not feel the negative effects of these chemicals, but if your child's detoxification systems are taxed, they may be affected. Small exposures over time add up. It's your job to remove as many of them as possible, especially if they are daily.

Installing a $100 carbon shower filter that you can order online is a great investment for your whole family. You'll find some links to affordable faucet and shower filters on the resources webpage for the book.

A Note About Swimming Pools

Swimming pools are highly chlorinated to stop the growth of algae and other organisms. Even standing near one means you're breathing in some chlorine. Not as much of a problem if you're healthy, but while you're still working on improving your child's wellbeing, it's probably best to avoid them. Otherwise, try to have them shower off immediately after getting out of the pool when going swimming.

Foods and Additives to Avoid

Let's summarise some foods and additives you need to try to avoid as much possible.

Common Foods to Avoid

Unfortunately, common knowledge is not common practice. We know certain things are not good for us or our families, yet we continue to buy them out of habit. The following are everyday items you need to minimise as much as possible (and ideally eliminate completely):

- Breakfast cereals (the popular ones in the supermarket)
- Fried foods
- Processed meats, sausages, and hotdogs
- Baked goods such as cupcakes, croissants, cakes, and others
- Junk food takeaways from popular fast-food chains
- Vegetable oils and spreads
- Sodas (including diet soda) and non-organic fruit juices
- Sugar, sweets, and store-bought cakes, deserts or puddings

E Numbers

E numbers are used to denote various food additives on ingredient labels in Europe and several other countries that use the system.

What many people don't know is that many of those innocuous-looking E numbers hide pretty sinister ingredients behind them.

Not all are bad, some are simply vitamins, plant extracts, or other organic compounds. For example, citric acid (E330) and malic acid (E296) are harmless additives used as acidity regulators. But you know what? Manufactures often use their full names on ingredient lists, rather than the E number, because people have become so wary of E numbers on labels.

Many E number additives contain aluminium, chlorine, formaldehyde, or other harmful chemicals. You may even see propionate (discussed in Chapter Three) used as preservative under the following numbers:

- E280 - Propionic acid
- E281 - Sodium propionate
- E282 - Calcium propionate
- E283 - Potassium propionate

As a general rule, if a product has E number ingredients, you're probably better off staying away from it, if you can. It often means you're buying a processed food.

Now, that is within reason, of course. I've seen certified organic beef mince with E300, E325, and E330 on the label. I searched for those numbers on my phone in the store, and saw that they represented vitamin C, sodium lactate, and citric acid. Being the geek that I am, I quickly checked what sodium lactate is in more detail. After seeing that it's generally harmless, I purchased the beef. But only because a better-quality alternative was out of stock that day.

I'm not saying you need to do this every time, but occasionally taking a deeper interest in what really is in your food will pay dividends for your family down the line. That way you will avoid the worst of the worst of food additives. Stay curious.

As a quick reference, the categories of E numbers are as follows:

- **E100 to E199** are reserved for food colourants
- **E200 to E299** are reserved for preservatives
- **E300 to E399** are reserved for antioxidants and acidity regulators
- **E400 to E499** are reserved for thickeners, stabilisers, and emulsifiers
- **E500 to E599** are reserved for acidity regulators and anti-caking agents

- **E600 to E699** are reserved for flavour enhancers
- **E700 to E799** are reserved for antibiotics
- **E900 to E999** are reserved for glazing agents, gases, and sweeteners
- **E1000 to E1599** are reserved for additional additives

Salt and Sweeteners

I won't belabour the point of reducing salt, sugar, and high-fructose corn syrup intake. By following my recommendations to cook your meals from scratch and minimise processed junk, you will make great strides in this area.

Just keep the following tips in mind:

- Throw out your table salt and replace it with quality sea salt
- Use stevia, xylitol, or decent quality honey as sweeteners when needed
- Keep an eye out for hidden sugar under these names: sucrose, dextrin, dextrose, malt syrup, palm sugar, brown rice syrup, corn syrup, HFCS
- If your child has certain gut issues or sensitivities (e.g. to FOD-MAPs), avoid inulin and sugar alcohols such as mannitol (E241), sorbitol (E420), isomalt (E953), maltitol (E965), lactitol (E966), xylitol (E967), and erythritol (E968)

While we're on the topic, let's talk about artificial sweeteners. The most common ones include:

- Aspartame (NutraSweet, E951, E962)
- Acesulfame potassium-k (E950)
- Saccharin (E954)
- Sucralose (Splenda, E955)
- Neotame (E961)
- Advantame (E969)

Do your best to steer clear of these. Not only is animal research linking many of them to cancer, but artificial sweeteners stimulate hunger and appetite, and encourage sugar cravings and sugar dependence.[5] This is precisely what you want to avoid when trying to get your child accustomed to a whole foods diet.

MSG and Other Excitotoxins

MSG, glutamate-based flavour enhancers, and other excitotoxins can be hidden in food under various names, so you need to remain vigilant when shopping. Some of the most common names include:

- E620, E621, E622, E623, E624, E625
- Glutamic acid (or anything with glutamate or diglutamate in the name)
- Natural flavourings
- Hydrolysed vegetable protein
- Hydrolysed protein
- Hydrolysed plant extract
- Plant protein extract
- Sodium caseinate
- Yeast extract
- Texturised protein
- Autolysed yeast
- Hydrolysed oat flour
- Calcium caseinate
- Malt extract, malted barley, or other malted ingredients
- Soy sauce, soy protein, or soy extract

Emulsifiers

Emulsifier use is widespread in the food industry, as I touched on in Chapter Five - from baked goods and desserts, to condiments and beverages. Frequently used ones to keep an eye out for include:

- Mono- and di-glycerides (E471), and derivatives
- Sodium aluminium phosphates (E541)
- Lecithin
- Stearoyl lactylates
- Polyglycerol esters (PGE)
- Polyglycerol polyricinoleate (PGPR)
- Sorbitan esters
- Sucrose esters
- Polysorbate

Preservatives

Examples of preservatives you need to steer clear of include:

- BHA (E320, butylated hydroxyanisole)
- BHT (E321, butylated hydroxytoluene)
- Propyl paraben (E216) and other parabens (E214, E218)
- Propyl gallate (E310)
- Nitrates and nitrites (E249, E250, E251, E252)
- Sodium benzoate (E211)

Most of the above are suspected to be implicated in cancer or to be endocrine disruptors, so it's best if you avoid them altogether. For example, BHA is anticipated to be cancer-causing based on evidence from animal studies.[6]

Sodium benzoate and some artificial colours have been shown to cause hyperactivity in children.[7] That's even at the concentrations normally found in foods.

During the writing of this book, I needed some sleep support to help me switch off my brain after 12 hours at the computer every day for months on end. I went to a health store and was shocked to see how many products intended to aid sleep contained preservatives and artificial colours! You get your valerian, passionflower, and melatonin along with substances that can have the exact opposite effect. How ridiculous is that?! Naturally, those products were the cheapest on offer. As the old saying goes - you get what you pay for.

Food Colourants

As mentioned in the previous section, some food colours have been shown to cause hyperactivity in children.[7] If you research artificial food colourants, you will discover that many synthetic or petroleum-based ones eventually get banned for use in food and drinks. That should make us uncomfortable to have any currently approved ones in the products we buy.

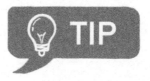

When reading food labels, keep in mind that E100 to E199 numbers are reserved for colourants. If you see numbers within that range on a product you're considering buying, at least give them a quick search on your phone to ensure they are not synthetic colours.

Examples of artificial food colourings to avoid include:

- Tartrazine (E102)
- Sunset Yellow FCF (E110)
- Erythrosine (E127)
- Allura Red (E129)
- Patent Blue (E131)
- Brilliant Blue (E133)
- Brilliant Black (E151)

Avoiding Other Toxins

After tackling the most important issue, namely that of toxins in the food you feed your child, the next challenge is addressing their immediate environment. Again, easier said than done in a world where we're drowning in plastics and chemicals.

As we discussed in Chapter Five, sources of harmful exposure are widespread, insidious, and too-often, seemingly innocuous. Some examples include:

- Plastics in bottles, food packaging, toys
- Flame retardants in furniture, carpets, beds, and children's clothes
- Cleaning materials
- Petroleum-based products
- Cosmetics

- Paper receipts
- Detergents
- PVC floors and pipes
- Building materials
- Garden products
- Pet shampoos and lice or tick sprays

Generally, anything that is produced using industrial manufacturing processes is likely to have toxic compounds in it. These can include solvents, synthetic rubber, glues, resins, and literally hundreds of other chemicals.

Let's consider some of the above and ways to reduce your child's exposure.

Plastics

Some tips to reduce your use of plastics:

- Replace your plastic containers and bottles at home for glass or metal ones.
- Replace plastic cooking utensils with wooden or metal alternatives.
- Replace plastic chopping boards with wooden ones.
- Never heat plastics in the microwave (never use the microwave, unless you have no other option).
- Try to avoid canned foods (many cans are lined with plastic)
- Avoid food and drinks served to you in plastic, especially if they are hot.
- Replace cling-film and aluminium foil with paper wrap alternatives.
- Try to avoid PVC or vinyl mattress covers - instead opt for natural cotton with a polyurethane laminate (PUL) or polyethylene layer.
- Avoid plastics with the recycling symbols 3, 6, and 7 as they may contain BPA, phthalates, and other harmful chemicals. Plastics with symbols 2, 4, and 5 are better alternatives. Products made using polyamine, polypropylene and polyethylene are also generally safer.

AVOID:

V/PVC PS OTHER

SAFER ALTERNATIVES:

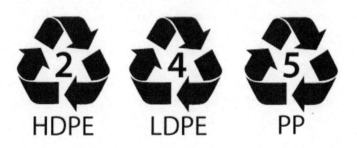

HDPE LDPE PP

Pots and Pans

After replacing your plastic cooking utensils with wooden or metal ones, you want to throw away your non-stick and aluminium pots and pans responsibly. Replace them with stainless steel, cast iron, or ceramic versions. If you must, gradually replace them one-by-one, starting with the pot or pan you use most often.

Cleaning Products

We've been terrified and brainwashed to think that unless we use the cleaning products marketed to us, we're leaving our floors, toilets, and kitchen counters filthy and dangerous.

But not only can you buy cleaning products from health stores that are made from safer ingredients, you can even make your own using nothing more than baking soda, lemon juice, and vinegar. Add in a few drops of essential oils for fragrance and you have most bases covered.

So, please do your whole family a favour and throw out all the conventional harsh cleaning supplies you have and replace them with gentler substitutes. This includes all products for dishes, windows, floors, counters, toilets, and bathrooms.

The same goes for antibacterial soaps - natural and organic soaps do the cleaning job just as well, without the harmful chemical residues.

While you're at it, replace your laundry detergent and fabric softener. They are full of toxic chemicals that your child can inhale or absorb through their skin. Your local health store should have much better alternatives.

Cosmetics

Children don't need much, if any, cosmetic products, but remember that you set the example for your child for later in their life. So, please think about what example you want to set for them and consider making positive changes to your own personal health, hygiene, and beauty regimes.

The common products we can buy in the department store are loaded with phthalates and other chemicals: skin care products, perfumes, shampoo, nail polish, creams, and after-shave lotions. Many conventional antiperspirants contain aluminium, so make sure you buy yours made from organic ingredients.

The EWG's Skin Deep database could help you in this regard. Search for the products you use regularly there to see if any are particularly toxic. You might be surprised what you find. I sure was. Since then I have used pretty much no face creams or washes, after-shave, or other "self-care" products. I also make sure all shower gels, shampoo, and soaps we buy in our home are as gentle and safe as possible.

Pesticides and Garden Products

Be wary of insecticides in spray cans and any garden chemicals you purchase and use. Many pesticides, herbicides, and artificial fertilisers are available that contain chemicals you want nowhere near your child, no matter their state of health.

Pet Products

Standard pet shampoos and delousing sprays contain toxic chemicals that would make your head spin. A big risk is you washing or spraying your dog, then your kids playing with it and getting the chemical residues on their hands.

It's best to seek out pet shampoos made from natural ingredients and make sure that you rinse your dog or cat thoroughly after spraying them for lice or ticks. Always err on the side of caution with this, especially if your child loves to play with the pet and is on the younger side.

Building Materials

It's hard to keep your kids away from building materials when you live in a building, but you can minimise your use of them. There are also companies offering non-toxic paint and renovation supplies. I would advise you to do a cursory Internet search next time you need to do a job around the home and purchase the safest products you can find. You certainly do not want your child breathing in fumes from conventional paints or finishes.

New Furniture

When shopping for new furniture or beds, look for items that have no added flame retardants.

If at all possible, allow new carpets and furniture such as couches or mattresses to off-gas away from your family for at least several days before bringing them inside the home. Longer if possible. If you can keep them on a balcony or in the garage and away from everyone, it would be ideal. If you don't have the extra space, putting them in a ventilated room that is used the least by your family is your next best option.

Sunscreen

Standard sunscreens have ingredients that will make anyone cringe after they do some research on them. The EWG's Guide to Sunscreens is a resource that can help you find the right product.

Some tips for which I credit the EWG include to never buy:

- Spray sunscreens and bug-repellent-and-sunscreen combo spray
- Any sunscreen with SPF higher than 50
- Products that contain retinyl palmitate, retinol, vitamin A, oxybenzone (benzophenone-3), or fragrance as an ingredient

Products with zinc oxide or titanium dioxide are safer options.

Dental Products

Find fluoride-free toothpaste and ask your dentist to not use fluoride products when working on your child's teeth. Most health stores carry fluoride-free toothpaste. Also, make sure that your child never gets mercury fillings.

Improving Your Home's Air Quality with a HEPA Air Purifier

Here's a quick but valuable tip to finish off this chapter: buy a HEPA (high-efficiency particulate absorbing) air purifier for your home and consider purchasing a smaller unit for your child's bedroom.

HEPA air purifiers improve the air quality in your home and reduce dust, pollen, pet dander, mould spores, and other allergens. You can get a decent quality unit for $50-$150 on Amazon. It's a worthwhile investment - you can really feel the difference in the air quality after having a unit run for an hour. Check out some of my recommendations for quality brands on the resources webpage for the book.

Wrap-up

In this chapter, we discussed strategies to reduce your child's toxic exposures. By now, you understand the importance of an all-organic diet. You understand how crucial it is to minimise all processed and junk foods, and the plethora of additives in them.

We looked at simple, but effective, ways to significantly reduce plastic residues ending up in your food. You saw how some relatively easy substitutions around the home can greatly diminish the chemical onslaughts on your child's detoxification systems.

Once again, I would encourage you to get acquainted with the EWG's resources and continue your education. We can only cover so much in one chapter, so when you have the basics mastered, try to take it to the next level.

CHAPTER NINE: IMPROVING SLEEP

Overview of This Chapter

You may find that once you improve the diet, remove inflammatory foods and additives, and add in the core supplements discussed in the next chapter, your child's sleep naturally improves. That is how powerful these seemingly simple interventions can be.

In this chapter, I'll show you how making some subtle changes to your child's sleep routine and environment can give you extraordinary results. Some of the tips and tactics I'll discuss may seem to be common sense, but they certainly are not common practice to many. Once you begin to implement them, you may be surprised how much your child's sleep improves.

Before we get into it, please indulge me in a brief review of the reasons why we even want to attempt to improve your child's sleep.

Let's preface the next section with this quote from a paper:

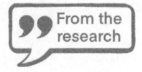

"Sleep problems may significantly influence the cause and/or exacerbate the core disease of ASD if left untreated."[1]

We'll have to forgive the use of the word "disease", especially when the authors' first language isn't English. But the take-home point is that sleep issues are more than likely going to contribute to poor health and even to ASD symptoms.

Sleep Problems in ASD

Sleep abnormalities are very common in ASD, with some 50% to 80% of children being affected.[2][3] The most prevalent sleep disorders are:[1][3-6]

- Difficulty falling sleep
- Increased bedtime resistance
- Frequent night-time awakenings
- Reduced sleep duration
- Morning rise problems
- Daytime sleepiness
- Sleep disordered breathing such as snoring, sleep apnoea, and mouth-breathing (I'll briefly cover breathing in Chapter Twelve)

Sleep deprivation can have serious health consequences, as you can imagine. Quality sleep is essential to support growth, the immune system, memory formation, healing, and brain maturation.[7-9]

Apart from complications with physical health, some studies have associated sleep disturbances with behavioural issues in ASD such as anxiety, aggression, and impaired social interaction and communication.[4][5][10][11]

Sleep problems can:[2][9][12-15]

- Contribute to inattention, hyperactivity, anxiety, and depression
- Exacerbate repetitive and stereotypic behaviours
- Contribute to aggression, defiance, and other challenging behaviours
- Interfere with learning, memory consolidation, cognition, communication and socialisation skills, and motor development

On the other hand, there is research demonstrating that improving the quality of sleep often translates to improvements in daytime behaviour.[16]

Let's not forget that if your child is not sleeping well, there's a high chance that you won't be sleeping well, which translates into poorer quality of life for both of you. In fact, research has shown this to be the case[17], even though we intuitively know it. Problematic sleep in autistic children has also been associated with higher levels of parental stress.[18-22]

I hope that by improving your child's sleep, you will also reap the benefits.

The Gut's Influence on Sleep Issues

Gut dysfunction is a significant contributor to sleep disorders, but this information seems to have evaded many practitioners for the longest time.[1]

Studies have shown that autistic children with gut problems tend to have a higher prevalence of sleep disturbances.[23-25] Gastrointestinal symptoms are also associated with insomnia and other sleep disturbances in autistic children.[26]

Many people know that the sleep-inducing hormone melatonin is secreted by the pineal gland (in the brain) at night, and that it helps us regulate our sleep-wake cycle. However, during the day, most of the melatonin production occurs in the wall of the gut. It's estimated that there is at least 400 times more melatonin in the gut than the pineal gland.[27] Do you see how leaky gut, inflammation, and pathogenic infections can have systemic repercussions for your child that may seem unrelated?

Strategies to Improve Your Child's Sleep

Addressing your child's sleep disturbances early in their life, and as quickly as possible, should be high on your priority list. One longer term study in Norway found that sleep problems in autistic children tend to remain even past mid-puberty[28] - a sign that these issues don't just resolve themselves with age.

Improved sleep will increase the likelihood of other therapies and interventions showing positive results, including those aimed at behaviour. As I like to say, if you improve the hardware, the software will function much better. Of course, one of the best ways to improve our hardware is to get quality, restorative sleep. It's indispensable, like charging your smart phone.

The good news is that a little education can go a long way. Research has shown that even a brief informational session on sleep for parents with autistic kids can have significant improvements on their children's sleep quality and behaviour.[29]

Let's discuss the most important basics around improving sleep hygiene and environment.

The Importance of Light and Dark During the Day

To maintain an optimal sleep-wake cycle, your home environment needs to emulate Mother Nature as much as possible. This means that your child needs to get a lot of daylight in the morning and throughout the day. The blue light from the sun helps to set a healthy sleep rhythm. When we are exposed to light upon awakening, our cortisol (a stress hormone) spikes to help us wake up and get going. We call that the cortisol awakening response (CAR).

If the CAR doesn't get stimulated properly for any reason, we can have difficulties with waking and during the day, such as drowsiness or low energy levels. This is why you want your child to wake up to bright daylight, if possible. Time spent in the sun every day is essential for health, so try to do some activities outside if you can.

Then, as evening approaches and the sun starts to set, you need to start reducing the light. Certainly, you want the lights turned down as low as possible at least one to two hours before bedtime. You will need to make sure all devices that emit blue light (TVs, tablets, phones) are turned off, because blue light at night disrupts melatonin production.[30]

Blue light can be particularly detrimental to autistic children as some of them may already be at risk for abnormally low melatonin levels.[31-36] Some researchers have even found correlations between levels of melatonin and autism severity,[34][35] meaning that the study participants with the lowest levels of melatonin tended to have more severe autism.

Sleep Environment

Your child's bedroom needs to be conducive to quality sleep. Unfortunately, our modern lifestyles are just the opposite. One study found that autistic boys (aged 8 to 17) who had a computer, TV, or gaming console in their bedroom, got less sleep than their peers who did not have those devices in their bedrooms.[2]

What does that result in? You have children that get less sleep that is also less restorative because of all the stimulation and blue light prior to it. In other words, to put it bluntly, electronic devices with screens have no place in your child's bedroom.

Some ideas to improve the sleep environment:

- The bedroom needs to be cool, quiet, and as dark as possible (if your child is not afraid of the dark).
- If you need to have some lighting in the room, consider red LED bulbs. Red light does not disrupt the human circadian rhythm as much as blue light.
- Put dark electrical tape (or similar) on LEDs and other lights that emit disruptive light at night.
- Better yet, turn off or completely remove all electronic devices from your child's bedroom.
- Keep the wi-fi router off at night, and as far away from your children as possible at all other times.
- Consider buying an inexpensive HEPA air filter to improve the air quality in your child's room, as well as to generate background noise that can help drown out other sounds.

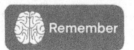

As a quick reminder, your child's bedroom needs to be free from toxic materials as much as you can help it. You simply cannot allow your child to breathe in toxic compounds from air fresheners, fresh paint, varnish, or new carpets, beds or furniture while they sleep.

Sleep Hygiene Summary

The core principles of sound sleep hygiene:

- Turn down bright lights at home one to two hours prior to bedtime.
- Turn off TVs, tablets and other screens one to two hours prior to bedtime.
- Avoid other overly stimulating activities before bedtime.

- Avoid sugary foods around bedtime, as they can cause blood-sugar fluctuations that can disrupt sleep.
- Design a bedtime routine that works for your family. It may include reading stories, Epsom salt baths, calming essential oils, or any other activities that work for you.
- Have a consistent sleep schedule. Display it prominently at home and point to it whenever your child resists bedtime, reinforcing the importance of rules.
- Try not to switch on the lights in the middle of the night, as this will disturb both your child's, and your own sleep rhythms. Again, consider purchasing some red LED lights for night-time waking to minimise sleep rhythm disruption.

Using Sleep Aid Supplements

In Chapter Eleven, I'll cover some supplements you can use to support your child's sleep. Supplementation and lab testing are the two areas in which I do the most research, so naturally I endorse utilising them intelligently in any health-building program.

However, I often reiterate that supplements won't salvage a lousy diet or lifestyle. They certainly won't provide the expected benefits if your child's gut is dysfunctional. What I see repeatedly is parents using melatonin to treat the symptoms. Their child is not sleeping, so they give them melatonin, and it works for a while. The problem is that they stop there and do no further investigation. What happens when the melatonin stops working? Back to square one, with pretty much no options (unless you consider pharmaceuticals an option). I'm not blaming them, of course. Most have not been taught the information you're learning in this book.

But as I stated at the beginning of the *Autism Wellbeing Plan*, symptoms are outer manifestations of underlying problems. We need to figure out what the hidden causes are and seek to address them. Treating symptoms is a futile game of whack-a-mole. You deal with one, another comes up. You suppress that one, more surface. You can't win that game.

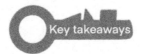

Key takeaways

What's the point I'm making? Sure, you can use supplements to help your child sleep better. But they should be used temporarily while you and your practitioner investigate and address the underlying causes of *why* your child is not sleeping well. You can also have them handy for times when your child needs extra sleep support.

But please, remember that there is always a cause (or several) contributing to any given issue which needs to be investigated in order to resolve it fully.

Wrap-up

In this chapter we covered the basics of sleep hygiene and making your child's bedroom as conducive to restful sleep as possible.

They were mostly simple changes but can be powerful when implemented in the context of the whole program. We'll now turn our attention to the core five supplements you can use to support your child nutritionally.

CHAPTER TEN: THE CORE FIVE SUPPLE-MENTS

Overview of This Chapter

The beauty of supplementation is that for relatively little effort you can provide your child with much-needed nutrients to support healing, growth, and development. In this chapter, we'll delve into the basics that should be part of almost every health-building program.

I'll start by summarising the rationale for complementing your child's diet with additional nutrients, regardless of how good it is. We'll then consider some important points to keep in mind when it comes to supplementation. The rest of the chapter will focus on the core five supplements:

- Digestive enzymes
- A multivitamin and mineral blend
- Probiotics
- Essential fatty acids
- Calcium and magnesium

I'll give you some details on each of them, including reasons for their inclusion in your child's program, their benefits, as well as tips for choosing the right ones.

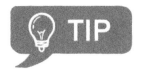

Selecting quality supplements can be challenging (especially if you're busy and are just starting out) and there's nothing worse than paying good money for a bad or useless supplement. That's why I've created a free video course to help you out. I will show you how to separate the quality products from the marketing hype and junk ingredients. You'll get a link to it in the welcome email after signing up to my mailing list. I hope it saves you some time, money, and stress.

The Rationale for Supplementing Your Child's Diet

There are many excellent reasons to supplement your child's diet. The most important ones to consider are:

- Self-selected and limited diets put children at risk for nutritional deficiencies and imbalances.
- Gut infections, oxidative stress, increased toxic burden, and other bodily stressors greatly increase nutrient demands.
- Dysbiosis in the gut may impair nutrient digestion and absorption.
- Today's food is much less nutritious than that of even 50 to 100 years ago.
- Nutrient supplementation has been shown in research to improve health biomarkers and even some autistic symptoms.[1-3]

A 2010 paper compared micronutrient supplementation against using medications in children with autism. While both groups showed improvement, the micronutrient group showed better improvements in autistic symptoms.[3] The authors also stated:

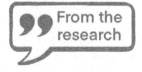

"There were some advantages to treatment with micronutrients - lower activity level, less social withdrawal, less anger, better spontaneity with the examiner, less irritability, lower intensity SIB [self-injurious behaviour], markedly fewer adverse events, and less weight gain. Advantages of medication management were insurance coverage, fewer pills, and less frequent dosing."[3]

Supplementation Considerations

Keep the following points in mind as you introduce supplements into your child's health-building program.

- Supplements are usually tolerated better with food, although certain ones may need to be taken on an empty stomach.
- Always start low and slow, then gradually build up to the required dose. Depending on the supplement, this process may take a week to a month.
- Always start one supplement at a time. That way, if your child has a reaction, you will immediately know what may be causing it.
- Liquids, chewables, and powders may work better with children who won't take pills (a common occurrence with younger kids).
- Chewables usually have extra ingredients to make them palatable that may be less-than-desirable, such as sweeteners. While not ideal, it is often a fair trade-off to support your child nutritionally until they learn to take capsules.
- Colours, flavours, and fillers may cause reactions - often more so than the actual nutrients or active ingredients. Monitor your child's reactions and switch to a purer product if your child doesn't tolerate a supplement with questionable additives.
- Quality and ingredients matter. If you don't know the various forms of vitamins and minerals, get some guidance from your

practitioner. They should be able to help you avoid wasting money on cheaply made products. We'll cover the most important points in this book.

- Don't hide supplements in food. Yes, adding powders and drops is fine, but you want to get your child used to the process of taking their supplements. Explain the importance of nutrients for health and that they are playing an important part in this by cooperating with you.

- Supplementation will not compensate for a bad diet. A clean diet is *the* foundation of the health-building program.

Let me emphasise that last point. Supplementation will not help you get away with a poor-quality diet. There too many chemicals and additives in non-organic and junk foods. The burden will be especially high on your child if their detoxification capacities are diminished due to prolonged exposure to toxins or oxidative stress.

Digestive Enzymes

Any time the intestinal lining is compromised, whether due to leaky gut, inflammation, gut pathogens, or all three, the intestinal cells' ability to secrete digestive enzymes can be diminished.

In fact, several studies with autistic children showed that a substantial portion of them had deficiencies in various carbohydrate-digesting enzymes.[4-6] In one of the studies, all the children who had enzyme deficiencies had loose stools or gaseousness.[4]

Digestive enzymes assist in breaking food down more fully, which reduces the risk of undigested particles entering the bloodstream, where the immune system may perceive them as foreign invaders.

Though research into digestive enzymes in ASD is limited, some studies have shown promising results. One 12-week trial noted improvements in socialisation (90% improved) and hyperactivity (80% improved), along with better mood, attention, digestion, and sleep.[7]

Another study found significant improvements in behaviour, emotional response, and gastrointestinal symptoms after three months of digestive enzyme supplementation:[8] The main behavioural changes the researchers reported were improvements in restricted repetitive behaviours and stereotypic behaviours.

To help you evaluate options when shopping, below is your quick primer on digestive enzymes:

- **Proteases and peptidase** break down proteins
- **Amylase and glucoamylase** break down starchy carbohydrates
- **Lipase** breaks down fats
- **Papain and bromelain** are plant-derived enzymes, from papaya and pineapple respectively, that help to break down proteins
- **Lactase** breaks down the milk sugar lactose
- **Invertase** breaks down sucrose (table sugar) into its constituents glucose and fructose
- **Cellulase and xylanase** help to break down plant cell walls and other tough-to-digest plant fibres
- **Phytase** breaks down phytate, which is a plant compound that binds with minerals and hinders their absorption (I briefly mentioned it Chapter Seven)

A few points to keep in mind:

- Your enzyme blend of choice should include a balanced mix of proteases, amylase, and lipase. Most brands include a mixture of a few other types of enzymes as well, but the main concern is to have the basics covered.
- Don't worry too much about the units of measurement (e.g. HUT, DU, AGU). Just make sure the important enzymes are at the start of the ingredient list. It means there's a larger quantity of them in the supplement.
- You can find chewable digestive enzymes. While these usually have added ingredients, the benefit of the enzymes will often outweigh some added flavours and sweeteners. Simply do your best to find the highest-quality products your budget allows.
- If your child reacts to (or doesn't like) chewables, or you want to use capsules for another reason, you can open up a capsule at the start of your child's meal and sprinkle its contents on the first few bites of food. Of course, the sooner you teach them to swallow capsules, the better.

Multivitamin and Mineral Supplements

A high-quality multivitamin and mineral can help fill nutritional gaps your child might have. Your supplement of choice should meet as many of the following criteria as possible:

- Includes the spectrum of B vitamins (B_1, B_2, B_3, B_5, B_6, B_9/folate, B_{12})
- Folate form is either folinic acid or methylfolate (not folic acid)
- B12 in its methylated form (methylcobalamin)
- Includes other vitamins (A, C, D_3, E, K)
- Essential minerals (calcium, magnesium, zinc, selenium, manganese, chromium).
- Trace elements (e.g. molybdenum, boron)
- No copper
- Adequate amounts of the nutrients
- High quality forms of the nutrients (e.g. chelated minerals, methylated B12 and folate)

We will discuss details related to some of the above points in this chapter and the next.

Probiotics

Probiotics are live micro-organisms, such as bacteria or certain yeasts, that can provide health benefits when taken in sufficient quantities. They can be helpful for your child in various ways. Probiotic research in autism is still relatively sparse, but we do have some evidence emerging that they can help to alleviate GI symptoms and, in some cases, even improve ASD symptoms.[9-13]

Taken into consideration with the large body of evidence from research on various other conditions, we have a strong case to use probiotics as a daily support for your child.

That is before we even consider the positive reports from parents and clinicians who have used them with autistic kids, of which there are many.

Probiotics can help to:[14]

- Reduce the overgrowth of pathogenic bacteria

- Improve constipation, diarrhoea, or other GI issues
- Positively modulate the immune system
- Reduce inflammation
- Produce antioxidants, vitamins, and other beneficial substances
- Stabilise the intestinal barrier
- Improve overall digestive health

A healthier, more stable intestinal barrier means fewer undigested food particles, toxins, and bacterial metabolites can enter the bloodstream and cause inflammation and immune reactions.

When searching for a formulation, look for one that includes as many of the below probiotic strains (we have the most research supporting their efficacy):

- Lactobacillus acidophilus[10][12][13]
- Lactobacillus rhamnosus[12]
- Lactobacillus plantarum[11]
- Lactobacillus casei[13]
- Lactobacillus delbrueckii[13]
- Bifidobacterium bifidum[13]
- Bifidobacterium longum/infantis[9][12][13]
- Bifidobacterium breve
- Saccharomyces boulardii

Additionally, if your child tolerates them, you can introduce fermented foods (in moderation) that contain probiotics:

- Sauerkraut
- Kimchi
- Kefir
- Home-made yogurt

It is best practice to take most probiotics on an empty stomach, either first thing in the morning or last thing at night. You need to make sure you give them to your child away from digestive enzymes and anti-microbials to maximise their effects.

One important caveat to keep in mind is that you should not start supplementing your child with probiotics if their immune system is compromised. Seek your clinician's guidance if that is the case.

Omega-3 Fatty Acids

Omega-3 fatty acids in the form of fish oil or cod liver oil can support the brain, gut, and help fight inflammation. Several clinical trials with omega-3 fatty acids have reported benefits for children with autism, including:[15-19]

- Significant increases in language and learning skills after 90 days[15]
- Improvements in autistic behaviour (on CARS, the Childhood Autism Rating Scale).[16]
- Improvement in essential fatty acid levels in the blood[16][17]
- Improvements in communication and social withdrawal[18]

Those trials were relatively short (up to 16 weeks), which is too short to observe the full effect of omega-3 supplementation. It takes about 6 months for levels in blood cells to reach a steady state,[1] however, the results are indeed promising.

High-quality cod liver oil is one of the best choices as it is easy to take in its liquid form and contains vitamin A and D. Intake and status of these nutrients can often be low in autistic kids, so this is a convenient way to add them to your child's diet. The fact that it is liquid allows you to control the serving size.

When searching for quality cod liver oil, you'll likely want some orange or lemon flavoured stuff, which will mask the fishy taste and smell, and help it go down easier. Be careful though, as cheaper products usually contain additives that you don't want. Try to find the brands which use the best quality ingredients and no artificial flavours or synthetic vitamins.

For example, when reading the supplement facts and ingredients list, make sure that the vitamin A and D origin is only from the cod liver oil itself, and not from retinyl palmitate or cholecalciferol. These are synthetic versions of the real vitamins A and D, respectively. Cod liver oil is actually closer to a whole food than a supplement, so you want to keep it as natural as possible.

More reasons to choose high quality fish oils:

- Polyunsaturated fatty acids like EPA and DHA oxidise more easily than other fats, so the manufacturing process must be of a high standard.
- Quality processes (such as molecular distillation) filter out heavy metals and pollutants.

Most kids will need 500-2000mg of omega-3s per day, depending on their weight. I cover how to select quality cod liver oil in more depth my free video course on choosing supplements for your child.

Calcium and Magnesium

We already addressed the fact that taking dairy out of your child's diet can greatly reduce their calcium intake. You also learnt that calcium can be protective against lead, and deficiency can increase lead absorption (which can have negative effects on cognitive and behavioural development).[20][21]

Magnesium is another important mineral that is often deficient in the diet, especially with kids who don't eat a lot of leafy green vegetables. It has a calming effect in the body and can help prevent or reduce excitotoxicity.[22]

Magnesium works synergistically with calcium. The two are best taken together at a 2 to 1 ratio (Ca to Mg), with a little vitamin D to help with calcium absorption.

In a nutshell, our rationale for supplementing your child with extra calcium and magnesium is:

- Taking dairy out of your child's diet may reduce their calcium intake significantly.
- Magnesium is critical to countless body functions. Diets are often deficient in it, and most children's multivitamins do not provide enough.
- Calcium and magnesium are sedative minerals (along with zinc). They can help relax the nervous system.
- Calcium and magnesium citrate (without vitamin D) taken with meals helps to bind oxalates in the gut.

When searching for quality forms of these minerals, keep the following in mind.

Calcium

High quality forms of calcium to look for:

- Chelated calcium, where the mineral is "attached" to an amino acid (e.g. look for "calcium amino acid chelate" on the label)
- Calcium citrate
- Calcium lactate
- Calcium ascorbate

Low quality forms of calcium to avoid:

- Calcium carbonate
- Calcium phosphate
- Dicalcium phosphate

- Tricalcium phosphate

Magnesium

High quality forms of magnesium to look for:

- Chelated forms, bound to amino acids (e.g. look for "magnesium amino acid chelate" or "magnesium glycinate" on the label)
- Magnesium citrate
- Magnesium malate
- Magnesium gluconate

Forms of magnesium to avoid:

- Magnesium oxide (poorly absorbed)
- Magnesium chloride (can cause GI distress)
- Magnesium aspartate, though a chelated form, may not be right for autistic children, as aspartic acid is an excitatory amino acid

It's difficult to take too much magnesium. Even if too much is taken, the body can regulate it. At worst, your child may have loose stools or diarrhoea.

In fact, this property of magnesium makes it a great remedy for constipation. Not all forms of it, though. Magnesium citrate would be the preferable option to try, after which you can try magnesium oxide.

Wrap-up

In my opinion, every child's diet should be supplemented nowadays, regardless of their health status. Children have to deal with an inordinate amount of toxins and food additives, yet our modern agricultural practises have depleted the soils from essential minerals. We are eating food that provides less nutrition even though we need it more than ever to protect ourselves from the toxic onslaught.

It's no wonder chronic disease rates are what they are and life expectancy in countries like the US is decreasing for the first time in decades. It's almost unfathomable, isn't it? Kids born today are expected to live shorter lives than their parents. If that doesn't shock us to the core, I don't know what will.

In the case of autistic children, the importance of regular comprehensive nutrient supplementation cannot be overstated. In this chapter, I showed you the basics you need to include in your child's program. There is much more we need to discuss, though, which is why we'll continue our supplements discussion in the next chapter.

CHAPTER ELEVEN: MORE ADVANCED SUP-PLEMENTATION

Overview of This Chapter

We'll now consider some more advanced supplementation strategies. First, I'll outline the supplements that can be useful for specific purposes such as supporting sleep, detoxification, or pathogen eradication.

Then we'll look at specific vitamins, minerals, amino acids, and other products that you can include in your child's program as needed.

At the risk of repeating myself, please allow me to stress the following. You may be able to start the supplements discussed in the previous chapter on your own. However, I highly recommend working with a clinician when introducing the ones I'll discuss in this chapter.

Nutrients are powerful. They work synergistically in some cases and antagonise each other in others. It's possible to create imbalances if you don't know what you're doing.

Also, remember that every child will respond differently to nutrient supplementation. Some will improve, which of course is our desired result. But others may not respond at all to the nutrient or may even get worse in some rare cases. You need someone who can take into account all the variables and help you course-correct should complications arise.

Having said that, the supplements we'll review are very safe, so there's no reason to be timid in including them into your child's health-building program. In fact, most of them are building blocks of the foods we eat. Simply remember that just like you wouldn't try to fix your car by yourself, there are dedicated professionals out there who can help you navigate this journey.

A few points to keep in mind:

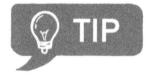

- It's a good idea to record dosages and details in your journal because it's easy to lose track.
- Keep note of your child's reactions as you introduce new supplements. Watch for changes in behaviour, hyperactivity, or sleep patterns.
- Follow the guidelines in the previous chapter and, as always, introduce each supplement one by one and gradually increase the serving amount.

Supplement Support for Different Purposes

Use this section as a cheat sheet on which supplements may be used for specific purposes. This is not a complete list, but it's a good starting point. Of course, your practitioner may recommend other suitable products.

Sleep

Supplements that can support restorative sleep:

- Melatonin
- 5-HTP
- L-Theanine
- GABA (gamma-aminobutyric acid)
- Glycine
- Taurine
- Calcium, magnesium, and zinc
- Vitamin B_6
- Epsom salt baths

Anxiety

Supplements to help with anxiety are similar to those that help with sleep, only you may want to take them at different times of the day.

- 5-HTP
- L-Theanine
- GABA (gamma-aminobutyric acid)
- Taurine
- Calcium, magnesium, and zinc
- Omega-3 fatty acids
- Chamomile, lavender, and lemon balm tea

You might want to have a few of the above stocked up just in case you need them. That way, as stressful situations come up (big day in school, moving house, sleepless night) you can be ready.

Gut Health

Supplements that can be used to support gut function and healing:

- Glutamine
- Probiotics
- Omega-3 fatty acids
- Digestive enzymes
- Colostrum
- Zinc or zinc carnosine
- Taurine
- Prebiotic fibre (in some cases)
- Aloe vera
- Glycine
- Collagen
- Mastic gum
- Deglycyrrhizinated licorice (DGL)

As an aside, bone broth is great for healing the gut. If you can make it or buy some, it's a great addition to a protocol.

Detoxification

Two of the best nutrients to support your child's detoxification system are the amino acids:

- Glycine (including DMG and TMG, discussed later)
- N-acetylcysteine (NAC), a source of cysteine

Both glycine and cysteine are required to make the antioxidant glutathione, which you know is needed to detoxify all kinds of toxic compounds, including heavy metals and chemicals.

If you provide your child with these amino acids, they will have a steady supply of "ammunition" to fight off the bad guys.

Other supplements that can be used to support detoxification include:

- Vitamin B$_3$ (niacin)
- Zinc
- Magnesium
- Selenium
- Glutathione (liposomal)

Using binders such as modified citrus pectin, zeolite clay, and charcoal can also help with "mopping up" toxins in the gut. Some modified citrus pectin products can also get into the bloodstream and help to bind and excrete certain heavy metals (more on this on the resources webpage).

Mitochondrial Function

The following supplements may be used to support mitochondrial function:

- L-carnitine and acetyl-L-carnitine
- Coenzyme Q$_{10}$ (ubiquinol)
- B vitamins (B$_1$, B$_2$, B$_6$, B$_7$/biotin, folate, B$_{12}$)
- Vitamin E
- Supplements that improve glutathione status (e.g. NAC)
- Alpha-lipoic acid

Pathogen Eradication

We'll discuss pathogen protocols in greater detail in the next chapter. For your reference, below are some herbs and supplements that can support pathogen eradication:

- **Anti-parasitic:** wormwood (artemisia), black walnut, berberine, goldenseal, garlic extract (allicin), oregano oil
- **Anti-bacterial:** berberine, garlic extract (allicin), uva ursi, olive leaf extract, oregano oil, caprylic acid
- **Anti-fungal:** grapefruit seed extract, garlic extract (allicin), olive leaf extract, uva ursi, caprylic acid, oregano oil, pau d'arco

Keep the following points in mind:

- Biocidin® is an effective combination herbal blend that comes in liquid form. The best part is that it tastes good, which makes it much easier to give to younger kids (I'll talk about it again in Chapter Twelve).
- Probiotics are an integral part of any pathogen protocol.
- N-acetylcysteine (NAC) can be used in pathogen protocols as it has anti-biofilm properties.
- Keep binders like charcoal or zeolite handy in case your child has a die-off reaction that is too uncomfortable (discussed in the next chapter).

Methylation

Supplements that can help support your child's methylation capacities:

- Vitamin B_{12} (methylcobalamin)
- Folate (methylfolate)
- Dimethylglycine (DMG)
- Trimethylglycine (TMG)
- S-adenosylmethionine (SAMe)

Antioxidants and Protection Against Oxidative Stress

Supplements that can help ameliorate oxidative stress include:

- Vitamin A, C, and E
- Magnesium and selenium
- N-acetylcysteine (NAC)
- Essential fatty acids
- Coenzyme Q_{10}
- Alpha-lipoic acid

Reducing Excitotoxicity

The following supplements can reduce excitotoxicity:

- Vitamin B_6 (pyridoxal-5 phosphate)
- Vitamin B_{12} (methylcobalamin)
- Vitamin C (buffered)
- Vitamin E (mixed tocopherols)
- Magnesium glycinate or lactate
- Zinc
- Coenzyme Q_{10}
- Acetyl-L-carnitine
- Alpha-lipoic acid

Correcting a Zinc-to-Copper Imbalance

The following nutrients can be used when correcting a zinc-to-copper imbalance:

- Zinc
- Vitamin B_6
- Vitamin C
- Manganese

Cognitive Function

Supplements to support cognitive function:

- Omega-3 fatty acids
- B vitamins (B_1, B_2, B_3, B_5, B_6, B_7, B_9, B_{12})
- Vitamin D
- Choline or choline-based supplements

Elevated Oxalates

Along with a low oxalate diet, increased water intake, and an anti-fungal protocol (when required), these supplements can help to address high oxalate levels:

- Calcium and magnesium citrate at mealtimes (to help bind oxalates in the gut and prevent their absorption)
- Probiotic
- Vitamin B_6
- Omega-3 fatty acids (fish oil or cod liver oil)
- Taurine
- Selenium
- N-acetyl glucosamine
- Chondroitin sulphate
- Vitamin E
- Arginine

Immune Function

Immune support supplements include:

- Vitamin A, C, D, and E
- Vitamin B_6, folate (B_9), and B_{12}
- Zinc
- Iron
- Selenium
- N-acetylcysteine (NAC)
- Glutathione (liposomal)
- Probiotics
- Garlic or garlic extract (allicin)

Vitamins

Beyond a quality multivitamin, there are certain vitamins that you can supplement individually.

Vitamin B12 and Folate

Vitamin B_{12} and folate are essential for methylation and glutathione metabolism. They are required to recycle homocysteine into methionine, which can be converted into other compounds required to support the methylation cycle.

A build-up of homocysteine is a blood biomarker for inflammation, so it's important to keep the cycle going by providing the supporting nutrients to your child.

Several studies have found vitamin B_{12} and folate to be beneficial for autistic children (in terms of improving biomarkers related to methylation and glutathione metabolism).[1-6] Some have even noted improvements in verbal communication and certain behaviours.[4][7]

These two vitamins are best taken together to prevent imbalances. Let's talk about each one in a bit more detail.

Vitamin B12

Vitamin B_{12} deficiency is common in people with digestive disorders. Blood tests may come back "normal", but that doesn't rule out a functional B_{12} deficiency, where the cells are unable to use the B_{12} circulating in the blood. The organic acids test (discussed in Chapter Six) has a marker for vitamin B_{12} (methylmalonic acid) that is a much better indicator of a deficiency than a standard blood test.

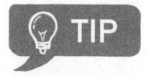

The best form of vitamin B_{12} to buy is methylcobalamin. A daily serving of 1000 micrograms is a good starting point.

There are several ways to give your child vitamin B_{12}:

- Liquid drops
- Sublingual lozenges
- Lollypops
- Intranasally
- Subcutaneous injections (best absorbed this way, but least practical)

The liquid form is the most convenient, especially when you get folate and B_6 in the same formulation. However, if you do have the means to use the injectable B_{12}, and your child tolerates this mode of administration, it is the optimal way to do it.

Folate

The two best forms of folate to use are:

- Methylfolate (sometimes written as 5-MTHF)
- Folinic acid

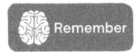

Folic acid, which is commonly added to cheap supplements, is the synthetic form of folate. It requires multiple conversion steps in the body to become activated and usable. Many autistic children have issues with making these conversions efficiently, so it's best to stick with the activated forms listed above.[1][8]

Depending on what your practitioner recommends, you can start with 400-800 micrograms per day, though much larger amounts have been used in some studies.

Vitamin B6

More than two dozen studies have been carried out on high-dose vitamin B_6 supplementation for autism, with most of them showing benefit.[9] In some cases, reported benefits have been quite remarkable, with improvements noted in communication, social interactions, behaviour, and intellectual functioning.

When I say "high-dose", we're talking about 25-100mg per day, sometimes even as high as 500-1000mg per day. Amounts this high are way over the recommended daily allowance but are still safe because B vitamins are water-soluble, thus excesses are excreted by the body easily.

Please note that your child does not need to be B_6 deficient to benefit from supplementation.

Vitamin B_6 is used to facilitate countless processes in the body, including:

- Production of major neurotransmitters (serotonin, dopamine,

GABA, and others)
- Needed for conversion of glutamate to glutamine
- Plays a role in glutathione metabolism
- Haemoglobin production (carries oxygen in blood)
- Gene expression
- Required for one of the enzymes that degrades oxalate in the body

Vitamin B6 comes in several forms. The two most common are:

- **Pyridoxine HCL** is the inactivated form, there is a metabolic step the body needs to do to make it usable.
- **Pyridoxal-5-Phosphate** (PLP, or P-5-P) is the activated form that the body can use directly.

Most of the research in ASD has been done with pyridoxine HCL, with about 4-8mg per kilogram of bodyweight (8-15 mg per pound), up to a maximum of 1000mg per day. If you don't notice much improvement with pyridoxine HCL, you may then consider trying PLP, or a mix of both.

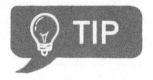

Always give vitamin B6 to your child with magnesium - about half as much in milligrams as the vitamin B6 amount. For example, for a 20kg (44 lbs) child, you could work up to about 350mg of vitamin B6 and 175mg of magnesium per day. (Note that you don't necessarily have to go this high if you see benefit from half the amount, for example.)

Magnesium enhances absorption and reduces hyperactivity, which is occasionally noticed in a small subset of children who take vitamin B6. Some supplement brands combine B6 and magnesium for convenience.

Try to spread out the servings over the day if possible, rather than give it all at once. Even if you can only manage two servings a day, it would be better than taking it all at once. A reasonable approach is to start with 0.5mg per/kg (1mg/pound) of vitamin B$_6$ and gradually increase the amount. Of course, these are just best practises, so please always follow your practitioner's advice.

Vitamin D

There is promising research showing that vitamin D supplementation can help autistic children. One notable study found significant improvement in autistic symptoms after three months of supplementation, as measured on the CARS and ABC (Aberrant Behaviour Checklist).[10]

Another study found that supplementation with vitamin D showed improvements in irritability, stereotypic behaviour, social withdrawal, and hyperactivity.[11]

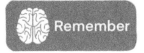
Remember

Vitamin D is a fat-soluble vitamin, meaning that it can accumulate in the body. That is why it is best to know your child's vitamin D status before deciding to supplement with it.

Minerals

Supplemental minerals come in many forms, some of them better than others. As I mentioned in the previous chapter, chelated minerals (attached to amino acids) are usually the best choice, because they are better absorbed in the body (are more bioavailable).

Zinc

Apart from helping to correct your child's zinc-to-copper ratio, zinc supplementation has many other benefits, including boosting immunity, and supporting growth and brain function.

One study found that daily supplementation with 1mg per kilogram of body weight plus 15-20mg helped to improve zinc status, lower copper levels, and improve cognitive-motor performance and CARS scores (a measure of autism severity).[12]

Another group of researchers found that severity of symptoms decreased in autistic individuals following zinc and vitamin B_6 therapy with respect to awareness, receptive language, focus and attention, hyperactivity, tip toeing, eye contact, sound sensitivity, tactile sensitivity, and seizures.[13]

The same research group found that autistic children with gastrointestinal issues significantly improved with respect to hyperactivity and stimming after zinc therapy, while those without GI problems did not improve in these symptoms.[14] This tells us that zinc supplementation could be especially helpful for children with gut issues.

In research outside of ASD, zinc has been shown to improve the growth rate in zinc-deficient children with mild-to-moderate growth failure.[15]

There are many forms of zinc, some of which are available as liquids and may be more convenient for you to give to your child. The best forms to use are:

- Chelated zinc (bound to amino acids, such as zinc glycinate, bisglycinate, or zinc methionine)
- Zinc acetate
- Zinc gluconate
- Zinc sulphate
- Zinc citrate

Stay away from zinc oxide and other forms not on the above list, just in case. You don't want to waste money on poorly absorbed supplements. When in doubt, ask your practitioner for guidance.

Iron

Iron should only be supplemented if your child's levels are low, as too much can be harmful. Low iron is more common in children under five years old, which makes it even more important to monitor your child's levels if they fall into that category. The best thing to do is have your practitioner run an iron test that also includes the marker ferritin on it.

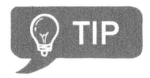

Supplemental iron is best absorbed when taken with vitamin C from a supplement or organic orange juice.

Selenium

It may be beneficial to supplement your child with extra selenium, even if their multivitamin and mineral supplement contains some. A blood or hair test should be able to inform your practitioner whether extra supplementation is prudent. Researchers have found selenium to be low in autistic children, so it's important to test for this essential mineral.[16-18]

Among many other roles in the body, selenium can help to:[16][19]

- Bind and excrete toxic metals such as mercury, lead, and cadmium
- Keep antioxidant enzymes functioning

As with most other minerals, you want a chelated form of it. Selenomethionine is the most common one you'll see.

Epsom Salt Baths (Sulphate)

As we've already covered, sulphation is often impaired in autistic children.[8][20-25] Because sulphate is poorly absorbed in the gut, Epsom salt (magnesium sulphate) baths are an effective and relatively easy way for you to improve your child's sulphate status.

All that you need to do is give your child a 20 minute warm bath, 2 to 3 times a week, with 2 cups of Epsom salt and half a cup of baking soda (which helps to increase absorption).[20] Remember that filtered bath water will reduce the chlorine and other harmful chemicals contained in it.

Other ways to supplement your child with sulphur or sulphate include using NAC or MSM, both of which we'll discuss shortly.

Lithium

Lithium is not classified as an essential mineral, but many clinicians have had amazing results with it, not just in ASD but also bipolar disorder, depression, and schizophrenia.

Data from animal studies and other research indicates that lithium may be an essential nutrient that plays a role in vitamin B_{12} metabolism.[26]

Studies have found hair or blood lithium to be low in autistic children.[8][16][27] One study found lower lithium in hair to be associated with more impairments in relating to people, emotion, adaptation to changes, visual response, and higher CARS scores (i.e. higher autism severity).[16]

Another study also tested the children's mothers and found lithium also to be low in the mothers of the children that had low hair lithium.[27]

Your child's hair or blood levels do not necessarily need to be low in order to give lithium a try. However, please consult with your practitioner before you begin supplementing with it.

Amino Acids

Amino acids are the building blocks of proteins such as hormones, neurotransmitters, enzymes, organs, and muscles. There are 20 dietary amino acids that we get from food or make inside our bodies. Essential amino acids are those that the body either can't make, or it can't make in sufficient quantities to meet demand.

Conditionally essential amino acids are those that we can make ourselves, but they become essential during times of illness, injury, or other stress. Many of the amino acids we'll review tend to be low in our diets, so supplementing with them can give your child a much-needed nutrient boost.

You can buy most amino acids in powder form. This makes them easy to mix into drinks and to control the serving size.

NAC

NAC (usually written as N-acetylcysteine or N-Acetyl-l-cysteine) provides cysteine, which is a precursor to the antioxidant glutathione. Cysteine, while found in small amounts in protein-containing foods, is most often the rate-limiting step in glutathione synthesis. This means that if your child's diet doesn't provide enough cysteine or glutathione demand is so high that cysteine is used up, then glutathione cannot be as readily made as it is needed.

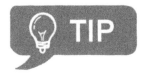

Supplementing your child's diet with extra cysteine via NAC is a great way to provide building blocks for the detoxification pathways.

Some ways you would know if NAC may be useful to include in your child's program:

- The NAC marker on the organic acids test (OAT) is abnormally low (N-Acetylcysteine Acid).
- The glutathione markers on the OAT are elevated (discussed in the next chapter).
- Your child has gut dysbiosis, or a compromised immune system.
- You have test results showing increased heavy metal or chemical burden, inflammation, or other markers that may indicate increased oxidative stress.
- Your practitioner recommends it based on their assessment of your child's unique case.

NAC has been shown to be effective in improving irritability and social functioning in clinical trials with autistic participants.[28-30]

Potential benefits of supplementation include:[31-33]

- Provides building blocks for glutathione synthesis
- Is an antioxidant in its own right
- Binds some metals and toxins directly
- Contains sulphur, so can help replenish sulphate
- Has anti-inflammatory properties
- Can help regulate brain glutamate levels
- Has anti-biofilm properties

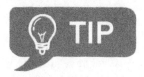

The most economical way to purchase NAC is in powder form, though you can also get it in capsules. The powder has a strong taste and smell, so you might need to mix it with acidic or sour juices such as lemon, orange, or other fruits in order to mask the taste.

Depending on your child's weight and your practitioner's recommendations, you may decide to supplement in the range of 900-2700mg per day over two or three servings, if possible.

Glycine

Glycine is the simplest amino acid and is also a neurotransmitter. It has many roles in the body, including:

- Part of the glutathione molecule (along with cysteine and glutamate).
- Binds toxins so they can be excreted safely.
- Makes up one-third of collagen and is important for protein synthesis.
- Precursor for many vital compounds in the body (e.g. creatine, haem).

- Plays a role in digestion and absorption of fats.

The best sources of glycine are animal foods that contain collagen such as chicken skin and joints (from healthy animals). Given how difficult it can be to get kids to eat foods like that, it makes sense to supplement with it, even if it's only a gram or two per day.

Research in adults with doses of 3-5 grams has shown sleep improvement benefits.[34-36] Naturally, if you want to give it a try, you would use less for your child.

Glycine powder has a sweetness similar to sugar, so you can add it to drinks or even sprinkle it on food without ruining the taste.

DMG and TMG

Dimethylglycine (DMG) and trimethylglycine (TMG, also called betaine) are basically glycine molecules with two and three methyl groups attached to them, respectively. They are methyl donors that can be used to support methylation in the body. Both go well with vitamin B_{12} and folate.

DMG and TMG are available in capsule or powder forms. Powder form is convenient as it can be mixed with other supplements and dosages can be controlled precisely. Common daily serving amounts are 500-1000mg, always starting low and gradually increasing the dose.

Without any lab tests, it's difficult to determine which of the two supplements is best suited for your child. In such cases, your best bet is to start with DMG and folate. If you see no benefits or you notice hyperactivity, try TMG. If you decide to give TMG a try, it is a good idea to give your child some taurine (250-500mg per day) prior to beginning supplementation.

Running some lab tests can help your practitioner make a more informed decision. One relatively simple way is to get your child's blood homocysteine level checked. If it is low, try DMG first. If it is elevated, TMG may be a better option.

GABA

GABA (gamma-aminobutyric acid) is a calming (inhibitory) neuro-transmitter that can be used to support sleep and reduce anxiety. It is made from the excitatory neurotransmitter glutamate, though there is often a failure to make the conversion in autistic children, as we covered in Chapter Four.

L-Theanine

L-theanine is a non-essential amino acid found in certain teas such as green tea. It has a similar structure to GABA and has a relaxing effect without being sedative. This means it may help with anxiety and stress, and can be taken at all times during the day without making your child drowsy.

Glutamine

Glutamine is a conditionally essential amino acid found in high amounts in animal products such as meat, dairy, and eggs. It is the pre-ferred food source for the intestinal and immune cells, making gluta-mine beneficial for gut health and immune support.

Taurine

Taurine is an antioxidant amino acid-like compound that has many vi-tal functions in the body, including in the cardiovascular and musculo-skeletal systems. It has neuroprotective properties and can protect cells from excitotoxicity and oxidative stress.[37]

Taurine has been reported to be low in some autistic individuals,[38-40] so supplementation may be warranted in some cases. It is used to make bile salts, which we use to digest fats, so it could also act as diges-tive support for your child.

Dietary sources of taurine include meat and fish. If your child's diet is low in these foods, you may want to try adding it to the supplement program. Because it has an inhibitory effect on the nervous system, tau-rine may help with sleep or anxiety when combined with the dietary, environmental clean-up, and sleep hygiene recommendations covered in this book.

L-Carnosine

L-carnosine (also known as β-alanyl-L-histidine) is an amino acid that has antioxidant and neuroprotective properties. Some ways it can be beneficial include:[41][42]

- Supporting GABA neurotransmission
- Reducing inflammation and neurodegeneration
- Decreasing glutamate levels, inhibiting glutamate release
- Protects against oxidative stress by preserving brain levels of the active form of glutathione

L-carnosine also appears to have anti-convulsive effects, which means it may help protect against seizures.[41] Experiments have shown that L-carnosine can suppress acetaldehyde toxicity, protect DNA from damage, and reduce the harmful effect of propionic acid.[43] However, much of the research has been done in animals or in *in vitro* experiments (in test-tubes), so we can't yet assume all these benefits will be transferred to humans.

One double-blind, placebo-controlled study reported that L-carnosine supplementation improved core ASD symptoms and language (800 mg L-carnosine daily for 8 weeks).[41] The researchers stated:

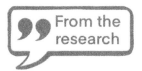

From the research

"The results of this study suggest that supplementation with carnosine can significantly improve receptive speech, socialization, and behavior in children with autistic spectrum disorders. These gains are observable both by parents and clinicians blinded to study group, as evidenced by the scores on the Clinical Global Impression."[41]

L-carnosine has also been trialled as an add-on to risperidone therapy in autistic children and appears to help improve hyperactivity and non-compliance.[42]

When you take into consideration that carnosine levels have been found to be low in autistic study participants,[44][45] we can build a strong case for at least giving this supplement a trial run.

Other Useful Supplements

In this section, I've included other supplements that you may find useful in your child's health-building program.

Carnitine

To recap our discussion from Chapter Four, carnitine is a nutrient that plays an important role in energy production. One of its core functions is to carry long-chain fatty acids into the mitochondria where they can be used to create energy. If you recall, it is often found to be deficient in autistic kids.

Two clinical trials with only carnitine found significant benefits for the children,[46][47] including improvements in CARS scores. Improvements were noted in concentration, eye contact, language development, and motor skills.[47]

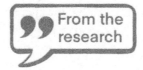

From the research

"In conclusion, the results of the present study suggest that L-carnitine therapy at a dose of 50 mg/kilogram body-weight/day over the course of three months of therapy significantly improved several clinical measurements of ASD severity. Further, there were significant correlations between increasing levels of serum free carnitine and several positive clinical outcomes among the study subjects examined. Overall, the L-carnitine therapy was well-tolerated."[46]

Other papers have also reported benefits from carnitine supplementation.[48] It is often used when a person has mitochondrial dysfunction.

The best sources of carnitine from the diet are beef and pork. The body can make it to a limited extent, but if your child does not eat much beef or pork, there is a higher risk for carnitine deficiency or inadequacy.

Carnitine from food is better absorbed than supplements (about 60% vs 15%), so a 125g (4.5oz) portion of beef will be roughly equivalent to 500mg of supplemental carnitine in terms of absorption.

There are two types of carnitine you will commonly find: L-carnitine and acetyl-L-carnitine. The body can convert one to another and we don't have much data on which is better, so it may be worth trying them in isolation and in combination.

However, to begin with, you can simply use acetyl-L-carnitine and think about combining them later. It crosses the blood-brain barrier more efficiently than L-carnitine, so may help to support energy metabolism in the brain.

A common practice is to supplement with 50mg-100mg per kilogram of bodyweight per day, spread over two servings, up to 2g. As always, the best strategy is to build up gradually to the full serving over a 2- to 4-week period.

Colostrum

Bovine (cow) colostrum is the first milk-like fluid from cows after they give birth. It's highly nutritious and contains various immune proteins as well as prebiotics, which feed the gut bacteria. It also comes in powder or liquid form, so it is easy to give to your child. Some key benefits of colostrum include:

- Helps to repair the gut and reduce inflammation
- Aids immune function and helps fight infections
- Provides much-needed nutrition (protein, fats, vitamins, and minerals)
- Promotes the growth of beneficial bacteria

There is a lot of anecdotal evidence of colostrum's efficacy in helping improve children's health, but the scientific interest is only beginning to increase.

A recent pilot study from 2019 investigated the benefits of colostrum and one strain of probiotic, and found that it was generally well tolerated. Reported benefits included:[49]

- Significant reduction of certain behaviours, including irritability, lethargy, stereotypy, and hyperactivity

- Increase in weight in chronically low-weight children
- Increase in appetite in some children and a willingness to eat new foods

Colostrum contains only a tiny amount of casein and lactose, but please bear the following points in mind when considering supplementing with it:

- Use colostrum only if your child has no strong casein reactivity
- Do not use colostrum if your child has a milk allergy or lactose intolerance
- Your best bet is to find casein-free colostrum, which is available on the market
- Quality matters - it is preferable to find organic and grass-fed sources

Ubiquinol

Ubiquinol is a form of coenzyme Q_{10}, an antioxidant that is used in our mitochondria to create energy. Supplementing with it can help during times of increased oxidative stress or mitochondrial dysfunction.

Your practitioner may recommend it if your child exhibits signs of mitochondrial dysfunction (discussed in the next chapter), or tests show increased oxidative damage (lipid peroxidation) or low total co-enzyme Q_{10} in the blood.

One group of researchers in Slovakia supplemented autistic children with 50mg of ubiquinol twice a day for three months, with benefits noted (including improved sleep and verbal communication) in a subset of the children.[50]

5-HTP

5-HTP (5-hydroxytryptophan) is a compound that gets converted to serotonin, which in turn can get converted to melatonin. Because sero-tonin plays a role in regulating mood and melatonin in regulating sleep, 5-HTP may be used to support both.

Please note that 5-HTP should not be taken with certain drugs such as anti-depressants (e.g. SSRIs), so make sure you consult with your practitioner before commencing supplementation with it.

MSM

Methylsulfonylmethane (MSM) is an organic sulphur compound that is found in tiny amounts in many foods. It is commonly used as a joint health supplement, but evidence is emerging that it can also help to reduce oxidative stress and inflammation.

You can use MSM to supplement your child with sulphate, as an alternative to Epsom salt baths. Any side-benefits beyond that are a welcome bonus.

MSM is a tasteless and odourless powder, so it can be added to drinks and mixed with other supplements. Daily servings size is commonly 500-2000mg, depending on your child's weight and sulphate level (if you have it measured).

Melatonin

Melatonin has been shown to be effective at improving sleep in autistic children.[51-57] It works particularly well when combined with cognitive-behavioural therapy.[57]

Melatonin helps the most with reducing time to fall asleep and increasing sleep duration. But its benefits do not end there. It also has antioxidant, anti-inflammatory, and neuroprotective properties.[58][59] Research is increasingly showing that melatonin has protective and healing properties in the gut, so you may get side-benefits when supplementing your child.

Some practical recommendations on how to approach melatonin supplementation:[60]

- Start with 0.5 to 1mg, 30 minutes before bedtime
- Increase by 1 mg every 2 weeks as needed, up to a maximum of 6 to 12mg
- Avoid over-the-counter formulations of melatonin that contain other active ingredients
- Consider "extended-release" melatonin tablets if your child has issues with staying asleep
- When your child's sleep cycle has normalised, wean them off the melatonin gradually, over a period of 6 weeks
- Capsules can be dissolved or mixed into filtered water, orange juice, or other liquids your child likes

SAMe

SAMe (also S-adenosylmethionine or S-adenosyl-L-methionine) plays a central role in the methylation cycle. The body makes it, but you can also get it in supplement form. SAMe can be used as a precursor to several important compounds, including glutathione and taurine. As a methyl donor, it supports countless essential processes in the body.

This is certainly one of the supplements where you need the help of a skilled practitioner to determine if it is right to use with your child.

Wrap-up

As you saw, most of the supplements we discussed in this chapter are found in the foods we eat (vitamins, minerals, and amino acids), or are derived from plants and herbs provided by Mother Nature.

We don't need much else to support health. You simply need to put back in what modern life has taken out and figure out what gaps in the diet or metabolism need to be filled (that's what the lab testing is for).

By now, you have the tools you need to effect amazing improvements in your child's wellbeing. We just have a few more topics to cover and loose ends to tie up. In the next chapter, we'll consider some practical aspects of designing and implementing your child's health-building plan.

CHAPTER TWELVE: PUTTING IT ALL TO-GETHER - YOUR AUTISM WELLBEING PLAN

Overview of This Chapter

Okay, we've laid the foundations, now it's time to look at how to struc-ture a health-building program for your child.

Remember, these are only guidelines. You need to seek the guidance of a knowledgeable practitioner and to continue to treat this infor-mation the way it's intended - as an educational resource. There are so many variables in every case, that it would be silly to think we could include everything you need to know in one book.

Here is a breakdown of the topics we'll cover:

- Start a journal
- Rule out potentially serious disorders
- Foundational lab tests: tips and key considerations
- What to do about pathogens
- Summaries of improving the diet, reducing toxic exposures, sleep hygiene, and supplementation
- Supporting toxin elimination
- Expecting challenges along the journey
- Monitoring your child's progress and re-testing
- An example initial protocol and sequence

Start a Journal

Step number one is to start a daily journal (if you haven't already) where you can record the many variables you will need to track, such as:

- Practitioner visits
- Tests run, results, and actions recommended
- Food intake
- Significant dietary changes
- Supplements started
- Your impression of the effectiveness of various interventions
- Behavioural changes
- Special events (e.g. "cheat day" due to a birthday party or Christmas dinner)
- Other useful data

Whether you use a physical diary, a Word document, or an Excel spreadsheet is entirely up to your personal preferences.

Rule Out Potentially Serious Disorders

Before you get into the details of specialised lab testing, dietary modifications, and supplementation you want to rule out any potentially serious conditions, such as:

- Gastrointestinal disorders such as inflammatory bowel disease (IBD), celiac disease, or gastritis
- Allergic disorders
- Mitochondrial dysfunction
- Breathing problems

This is not an exhaustive list. While I'll give you a few pointers here, you'll need to see to it that your doctor takes into consideration your child's health history when deciding what areas need further investigation. For example, epilepsy and seizure disorders are common in ASD, but are beyond the scope of this book.

Gastrointestinal Disorders

If your child has chronic gastrointestinal issues, it's a clue that you need to have their gut function examined by a specialist.

But how do you know if your child has gut problems? As we have discussed already, an underlying GI issue won't always be obvious, so you need to be aware of other ways gut discomfort can manifest in your child.

How to Tell If Your Child Has a Gut Issue

Clear tell-tale signs are the obvious ones:

- Constipation
- Diarrhoea
- Loose stools
- Visible pain or discomfort
- Direct verbalisations (e.g. child says "tummy hurts" or says "ouch," "ow," "hurts," or "bad" while pointing to abdomen)[1]

If your child is non-verbal or they have difficulties with communicating their pain or discomfort, it becomes increasingly important for you to be remain vigilant. This is where your journal may be a great tool to support your observations, but you also have your instincts as a parent. You know your child. You will be heightened to things that may seem "off" and can then investigate further with the knowledge you have gained in this book.

Other Physical Signs

Apart from the obvious clues, other signs of gut dysfunction may include:[1]

- Application of pressure to the abdomen: leaning tummy against or over furniture, pressing hands into it or rubbing it
- Any unusual posturing, which may appear as individual postures or in various combinations: jaw thrust, neck torsion, arching of back, odd arm positioning, rotational distortions of the torso, sensitivity to being touched in abdominal area, or flinching
- Facial grimacing or gritting the teeth
- Agitation: pacing, jumping up and down

- Unexplained increase in repetitive behaviours
- Mouthing behaviours: chewing on clothes (shirt sleeve cuff, neck of shirt, etc), pica (eating sand, soil, paper or other non-food substances)
- Constant eating, drinking, or swallowing ("grazing" behaviour)
- Frequent clearing of the throat, swallowing, tics
- Tapping behaviours: finger tapping on throat

Potential Behavioural Clues

The sudden emergence or worsening of the following can signal potential underlying gut problems:[1][2]

- Sleep disturbances (difficult to get to sleep or stay asleep)
- Irritability
- Aggression
- Self-injurious behaviour (e.g. biting, hits or slaps face, head-banging, unexplained increase in self-injury)
- Oppositional behaviour, non-compliance to requests
- Screaming
- Sobbing for no reason
- Sighing, whining, moaning, groaning

If you notice the above, but cannot recognise any clear environmental cause or influences such as unfamiliar events, change in diet, travel, or illness, they could serve as clues that an underlying gut issue could be present. In such cases, you may want to have your health care practitioner examine your child.

When to Go to a Doctor or Specialist

If you observe any of the below signs or symptoms, you should immediately contact your doctor to see if they recommend further testing and evaluation:[3][4]

- Weight loss
- A slowing down of linear growth
- Gastrointestinal blood loss (visible or on a stool test).
- Significant, chronic, or cyclical vomiting
- Chronic severe diarrhoea
- Persistent pain in the abdomen
- Unexplained fever

Additionally, if you have a family history of inflammatory bowel disease, or a doctor visit results in abnormal or unexplained physical findings, it is always best to err on the side of caution and ensure that serious conditions are ruled out.

Testing for Allergies

An allergy is an immediate immune reaction to foods or other particles, which is mediated by immunoglobulin E (IgE) antibodies within seconds or minutes of exposure to the allergens. As discussed in Chapter Two, they are often overlooked in autistic children and can cause serious distress.

Luckily, testing for allergies is relatively easy. Two common ways to test for them are:

- Skin prick or patch testing using small amounts of allergens, to see if any cause a reaction
- Blood testing to detect IgE antibodies

If any allergens are identified, you will need to steer clear of them as best as you can.

Mitochondrial Dysfunction

Some clues that your child may have mitochondrial dysfunction include:[5][6]

- You have a family history of mitochondrial disease
- Regression in your child's development, loss of skills
- Developmental delays
- Seizures
- Fatigue, lethargy
- Muscle weakness, exercise intolerance
- Ataxia (issues with movement or coordination)
- Motor delays
- Gastrointestinal abnormalities
- Cardiomyopathy (problems with the heart)

The more of the above that apply to your child, the more likely it is that mitochondrial dysfunction may play a role, and some investigative work on the part of your practitioner is in order.

Testing for Mitochondrial Dysfunction

In the next section of this chapter, we'll look at some markers on the organic acids test (OAT) that can indicate your child has mitochondrial dysfunction.

Whether you run the OAT or not, your doctor will probably want to run more in-depth blood tests to confirm mitochondrial dysfunction is indeed present. The following blood markers can be used as direct and indirect indicators.[5][7]

Direct markers of mitochondrial dysfunction:

- Lactate
- Pyruvate
- Lactate-to-pyruvate ratio
- Ubiquinone
- Alanine
- Alanine-to-lysine ratio
- Acyl-carnitine

Indirect markers of mitochondrial dysfunction:

- Creatine kinase (CK)
- Carnitine
- Aspartate
- Aspartate transaminase/aminotransferase (AST)
- Alanine aminotransferase (ALT)
- Ammonia

Some of these markers may be abnormal for other reasons. Or they may be in range, but it still may not be enough to rule out mitochondrial dysfunction. This is why this is an area where you need to work with a specialist doctor who may advise you to run other tests, such as urine amino acids, a skin or muscle biopsy, or a mitochondrial DNA test.

It has also been recommended by researchers to repeat abnormal tests, to verify that they are true abnormalities.[5] The human metabolism is highly variable, so any given marker can fluctuate considerably on a daily or weekly basis.

Breathing Problems

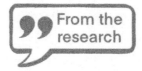

"Recently we have seen several studies published showing stronger data linking sleep disordered breathing in children to developmental and behavioral problems. Bonuck et al. demonstrated 40% and 60% more behavioral problems at age 4 and 7 years, respectively, in their long term outcome cohort study following children with parental reports of snoring, mouth breathing in sleep, and witnessed apnea. The behavioral problems seen were hyperactivity, anxiety, depression, and conduct disorders."[8]

Undetected breathing problems can cause your child significant discomfort and health complications. Some common ones include:

- Asthma
- Rhinitis, allergic (hay-fever) or non-allergic
- Sleep apnoea
- Adenoid or tonsil enlargement (hypertrophy)

Ideally, you want to identify and address the above (or other) issues as soon as possible. Not only do breathing problems contribute to anxiety and poor sleep, if left unaddressed they can have more serious health consequence over time.

That is because they may force your child to breathe through the mouth some or all of the time. Once mouth-breathing becomes a habit for them, other complications can manifest including altered face and jaw development, and crooked teeth.[8]

Researchers found that a history of sleep disordered breathing (snoring, sleep apnoea, mouth-breathing) in children up to five years of age was associated with 40% increased odds of the children having a special education need at the age of eight.[9]

In that paper, the researchers wrote:

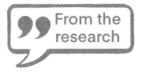

From the research

"...[sleep disordered breathing] is linked to delayed development, speech-language impairments, and adverse behavioral and cognitive effects."[9]

Another all-too-common issue is that of breathing too much. Also known as chronic hyperventilation, it is rampant in our society.

Over-breathing causes subtle, but important, changes in the levels of gases in our blood. It may surprise you to learn that breathing too much can actually reduce the oxygen that gets delivered to our tissues. That's because when we over-breathe (especially when combined with mouth-breathing), we expel too much carbon dioxide (CO_2). We need to maintain a certain level of CO_2 in the blood to assist the release of oxygen from the blood to where it is needed (in our cells and tissues).

Breathing too much (thus expelling too much CO_2) causes our airways and the smooth muscles around our blood vessels to tighten up (constrict). It can turn into a vicious cycle where we stay in a state of chronic over-breathing and reduced oxygenation of our tissues. Over months or years this can contribute to many health problems.

Why does mouth-breathing contribute to anxiety and poor sleep? The chief reason is because it activates the stress response, also known as the fight-or-flight or sympathetic nervous system. Allow me to illustrate.

Though I do not recommend that you try it (because it can make you dizzy), if you were to take 20 fast and deep breaths through the mouth right now you will feel that:

- Your heart rate goes up
- Your mouth dries up
- You become lightheaded

Now, clearly that is an exaggeration. It is certainly more subtle in real life, but you are starting to get the idea.

Try this now: close your mouth and breathe in and out through your nose 20 times as fast and deep as you can. The difference is night and day. It is really difficult to get the effect of mouth breathing.

To sum up the reasons you don't want your child to breathe through the mouth:

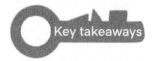
Key takeaways

- Contributes to anxiety, stress, or panic attacks (by activating the fight-or-flight nervous system)
- Reduces oxygen delivery to the body's cells and tissues, including the brain
- Contributes to poor sleep
- Can contribute to over-breathing (chronic hyperventilation)
- May worsen asthma, hay-fever, and non-allergic rhinitis
- Reduces exercise tolerance (kids "gas out" faster when breathing through the mouth)

What to Look For

The first step is always awareness. Signs of breathing issues to look for include:

- Does your child breathe through their mouth some or all of the time? Is it because of habit, a blocked nose, or other obstruction?
- Do they have other noticeable breathing issues such as snoring or holding their breath while sleeping (apnoea)?
- Non-allergic rhinitis: stuffy or runny nose, mucus, wheezing, sneezing, coughing. Usually triggered by something in the environment. Symptoms may be constant or intermittent depending on exposure to irritants.
- Hay-fever (allergic rhinitis): similar to non-allergic rhinitis but usually accompanied by watery eyes and itchiness of the nose, eyes, or throat. Usually seasonal and triggered by pollen.
- Asthma: shortness of breath, coughing, wheezing, chest tightness or pain.

What is Proper Breathing?

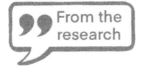

"When nasal breathing does not occur for any reason, the body is forced into a series of compromises that prioritize getting oxygen into our blood at the expense of the functions provided by the nasal breathing. Because oxygen is required for survival, we are forced to live with a host of acquired health issues as a consequence of chronic or intermittent mouth breathing. One such consequence, known as Sleep Disordered Breathing (SDB), is becoming pandemic in children, and directly affects their growth, development, intellect, academic performance, behavior, and much more."[8]

A healthy human breathes in and out through the nose all the time. It should be light, slow, and deep. Benefits of nasal breathing include:

- Slows down, moistens, filters, and helps disinfect the air coming into the lungs.
- Activates the "rest and digest" (parasympathetic) nervous system which has a calming and repairing effect on the body.
- Slows down the breathing rate and the heart rate.
- Activates and exercises the diaphragm, which also massages the organs around it.
- Keeps lymph flowing - aiding body detoxification.
- Increases production of the gas nitric oxide, which has many positive effects in the body including sterilising the incoming air and expanding the airways.
- Reduces loss of moisture (experienced when breathing through the mouth).

Benefits of Teaching Your Child Correct Breathing Habits

Improving your child's breathing is something you can do relatively quickly, at virtually zero cost. Your time investment can have many benefits for your child, including:

- Improved sleep
- Reduced anxiety
- Better oxygenation of the brain and other tissues of the body
- Improved concentration

Also, importantly, teaching your child proper nasal breathing as early as possible will promote the development of the jaw, face, airways, and straight teeth.

Using the Buteyko Method

The Buteyko Method (named after its creator Dr Konstantin Buteyko) is a series of easy-to-do breathing exercises and practises designed to reinforce health-promoting breathing habits. The most important tenets are:

- Always breathe through the nose (lightly, slowly, and deeply)
- Reduce chronic over-breathing (chronic hyperventilation)

The exercises are simple and easy to teach to children. All you need is some time and some tape to bring the lips together while doing them. The goal of the tape is to instil the habit of keeping the mouth closed, without covering the lips. It takes a few minutes to get used to it. While not all children will be comfortable with it, the easiest way to get them to wear the tape is when the whole family gets involved and carries out the breathing exercises together. This has the added benefit that everyone can improve their breathing habits whilst increasing time spent with each other and adding some fun to the mix.

The best resource I can direct you to is the Buteyko Clinic. Its director, Patrick McKeown, is a leading authority on the Buteyko Method and an expert on breathing. He has generously offered their complete Buteyko Method for children and teenagers program for free online at https://buteykoclinic.com/buteykochildren/.

If you feel that your child breathes through their mouth or has other breathing dysfunction, I would encourage you to take advantage of this valuable resource. It can even help with asthma and rhinitis (but don't forget to rule out issues such as enlarged adenoids to ensure there are no physical obstructions).

Please note that there are certain precautions and contraindications to using some of the Buteyko Method exercises (such as with children with type I diabetes or heart problems), so make sure you do your research if your child has any medical conditions. The Buteyko Clinic's website has all the information you need.

Foundational Lab Tests: Tips and Key Considerations

Testing takes times, which is why it's important to start organising it as soon as possible. Waiting for clinician appointments can take days or weeks. It can take up to a week for test kits to arrive. Timing the sample collection and courier pickup may take you a few extra days.

Then you need to wait for the lab to receive the sample, process it, and send the results back to your practitioner, who will need time to review them and set up an appointment with you. The whole process can take more than a month for some tests, especially if the lab is on another continent.

That is why you should not delay, because certain protocols and supplements can only be started after a test indicates they are necessary. Also, don't forget that waiting for the supplements can take a week or two.

In the rest of this section, I'll discuss some key considerations and points to keep in mind when you run the foundational lab tests.

Organic Acids Test

As I emphasised in Chapter Six, the organic acids test (OAT) is the most valuable test you can run for your child at the outset. It covers so many areas of the metabolism that it's extremely unlikely that you won't get some useful data to guide the design of your child's health-building program.

You need a clinician who knows how to interpret the OAT, of course, but the Great Plains Lab also includes their interpretation notes on the results. This is helpful for your practitioner because they will still be able to make sense of the test and act accordingly, even it's their first time looking at one.

Let's now take a look at some of the most useful markers on the OAT, and what you would do about them in most normal circumstances. The purpose of this is to give you a glimpse of the value the OAT has to offer and how a health-building protocol is designed. Naturally, your practitioner will consider the many variables that make up your child's case.

Yeast and Fungal Markers

If some of the following OAT markers are elevated, it is indicative of yeast overgrowth:

- Arabinose (indicates *Candida*)
- Tartaric (indicates *Candida*)
- Citramalic
- 3-Oxoglutaric
- Carboxycitric

We'll talk about the yeast protocol in the section "What to Do About Pathogens", coming up shortly in this chapter.

Potential Mycotoxin Indicators

When some or all of the following markers are elevated on the OAT, it may signal potential mould toxicity:

- 5-Hydroxymethyl-2-furoic
- Furan-2,5-dicarboxylic
- Furancarbonylglycine
- Tartaric

- Tricarballylic

The first four markers above are associated with *Aspergillus* mould, which is the most common mould we're exposed to in our environment and food supply. The fifth (tricarballylic) marker is associated with mycotoxins produced by moulds that predominantly grow on corn and some other grains.

If you find yourself in this situation, it's usually a good idea to run the MycoTOX test I mentioned in Chapter Six (check the resources webpage for more information).

Other markers on the OAT that can be used as clues include:

- Lactic
- Succinic
- Pyroglutamic

These markers can be elevated due to other reasons, so it's important for your practitioner to make correlations carefully and examine other potential contributing factors.

What are some physical clues that mycotoxins could be an issue for your child? Common mould exposure symptoms include:

- Fatigue
- Headaches
- Difficulty breathing
- Rashes
- Severe gastrointestinal distress
- Bleeding (e.g. nose bleeds)
- Eye pain
- Muscle or joint pain
- Pain on urination, bladder irritability
- Serious neurological or psychiatric symptoms
- Muscle weakness
- Problems with coordination or balance
- Mental fog, confusion

Keep in mind that smaller children can't verbalise many of the above symptoms, so increases in irritability, moodiness, or aggression can be a clue. Eye pain can be expressed as eye poking in some children.

We will discuss the protocol for mould in the "What to Do About Pathogens" section of this chapter.

Bacterial and Clostridia Markers

In most cases where pathogenic bacteria markers are high, you will want to address them with probiotics and a pathogen protocol (discussed later). Markers on the OAT that indicate bacterial overgrowth or a state of dysbiosis are:

- Hippuric
- 2-Hydroxyphenylacetic
- 4-Hydroxybenzoic

Clostridia Markers

The above are general markers of bacterial overgrowth or dysbiosis. If any of the markers below are elevated, it signals *Clostridia* bacteria overgrowth:

- **4-cresol** (*C. difficile*)
- **HPHPA** (*C. sporogenes, C. caloritolerans, C. botulinum,* and others)
- **4-hydroxyphenylacetic** (*C. difficile, C. stricklandii, C. Lituseburense,* and others)
- **3-Indoleacetic** (*C. stricklandii, C. lituseburense, C. subterminale,* and others)

If the test indicates that *Clostridium difficile* is present (by 4-cresol and 4-hydroxyphenylacetic), you have several options:

- Antibiotic treatment (e.g. metronidazole, vancomycin, fidaxomicin) and probiotics.
- Herbal anti-bacterial (e.g. Biocidin®) and probiotics.
- In some cases, and regions of the world, a faecal microbiota transplant (FMT) may be available to you. Ask your health care provider for more information on legality and availability in your area.

Your practitioner should advise you which option is most appropriate in your case. Generally, if your child has severe gastrointestinal and other symptoms, your provider may recommend antibiotics. On the other hand, if your child doesn't present with strong symptoms, you may wish to go the gentler and more natural route and use herbal antibacterials.

Mitochondrial Dysfunction

The following OAT markers may indicate mitochondrial dysfunction:

- Lactic
- Pyruvic
- Fumaric
- Malic
- Aconitic
- 3-Methylglutaric
- 3-Methylglutaconic
- 3-Hydroxyglutaric

As we discussed already, if your practitioner suspects mitochondrial dysfunction, it is usually best to get a more thorough evaluation to rule out any serious disorders. They may also recommend some supplements and mitochondrial co-factors outlined in the previous chapter to support your child's mitochondria.

Oxalate Markers

If the glyceric and glycolic markers are elevated, it can indicate genetic hyperoxaluria type I or II. These are rare conditions and, in such instances, a DNA test to confirm the disorder would need to be done.

Much more often, the oxalic acid marker is elevated, which can be associated with fungal infections or a high-oxalate diet. Oxalates can sometimes be elevated from supplementing with high doses of vitamin C.

When the oxalic marker on the OAT is elevated, the most common protocol to implement would include:

- A low oxalate diet (see Chapter Seven)
- Anti-fungal protocol if yeast markers are elevated
- Calcium and magnesium citrate at mealtimes (to bind oxalate and prevent absorption)

Your practitioner may also recommend some supplements listed in Chapter Eleven. A leaky gut increases absorption of oxalates, so it's important to focus on supporting its healing and repair.

Neurotransmitter Markers

As discussed in Chapter Six, the neurotransmitter markers on the OAT can be unbalanced due to various stressors.

It's your clinician's job to take into consideration your unique case and figure what may be contributing to the imbalances. Common culprits include bacterial infections (e.g. *Clostridia* and their metabolites), chronic inflammation, environmental toxins, and nutrient deficiencies. Sometimes, genetics may play a role.

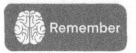

Certain foods and supplements can also cause elevations in the neurotransmitter markers, so you should not automatically assume the worst if your child's test shows an imbalance.

Indicators of Toxicity

When you see an elevation in the "succinic" marker on the OAT, it's a clue that your child may have some toxic exposure. It's a non-specific clue, which means it can be heavy metals or chemicals (and occasionally other factors such as nutrient deficiencies).

Other indications of increased toxic burden are when the following markers (for glutathione status) are elevated:

- Pyroglutamic Acid
- 2-Hydroxybutyric Acid

Or this marker (for the glutathione precursor NAC) is abnormally low:

- N-Acetylcysteine Acid

The best way to decide if further testing is needed is to take into consideration whether your child has been at risk for toxic exposure in the recent past, or in general.

If you've done a hair or other metals screening test, you will have more data with which to make a decision. For example, if the succinic marker is high and your child has elevated mercury and aluminium, we can suspect them to be playing a role in its elevation. If, however, heavy metal levels are low or normal, we may turn our attention to your child's environment. If you suspect chemical exposure, you may consider running a GPL-TOX or the Cyrex panel we covered in Chapter Six.

Along with ensuring your child's environment is as pristinely clean as possible, you will also need to support their detoxification systems with some of the supplements outlined in the previous chapter.

Stool Testing

Keep the following in mind when planning to run a stool test:

- If you're waiting for the test kit to arrive and haven't yet begun probiotic supplementation, wait until you collect the sample before starting the probiotics.
- If your child is taking probiotics, you need to discontinue them for 48 hours before collection.
- Some labs require discontinuing other supplements such as digestive enzymes or certain vitamins for some time before collecting the sample. Make sure you're aware of your lab's requirements.
- Depending on the lab, you may have to provide 2 or 3 samples, taken within a set period (e.g. 7 days) but separated by some time (e.g. 12 hours). This is usually the case for culture-based tests. DNA-based tests require only one sample, which adds to their convenience.

Up-to-date links to some quality labs and stool pathogen tests can be found at the resources webpage for this book.

Blood Testing

To recap what we covered in Chapter Six, the following markers should make up the basic blood tests you run on your child:

- Complete blood count (CBC)
- Comprehensive metabolic panel
- Zinc (in plasma)
- Copper (in serum)
- Iron and ferritin

- Folate and vitamin B_{12}
- Vitamin D
- Blood lipids (cholesterol, HDL, LDL)
- Thyroid panel (TSH, T3, T4)
- Homocysteine
- C-reactive protein (hs-CRP)

Of course, if your health care provider wishes to run more tests, all the better. They will take your unique case into account when making recommendations. More advanced testing can include:

- Serum carnitine (total and free)
- Serum ceruloplasmin
- Whole blood histamine
- Sulphate
- Micronutrient, fatty acids, and amino acids analysis
- Methylation profile
- Genetic single nucleotide polymorphisms (SNPs)
- Antibodies to various human tissues (e.g. brain and nervous system tissues, gut barrier proteins)
- Antibodies to various pathogens or their metabolites (e.g. viruses, Lyme's disease, LPS, mycotoxins)
- Antibodies to heavy metals and toxic chemicals
- Comprehensive thyroid markers

Naturally, any nutrient deficiencies or inadequacies need to be addressed. Similarly, if inflammation markers are elevated (homocysteine and hs-CRP), your practitioner needs to do some detective work to figure out what factors are causing the inflammation and address them. Thankfully, the rest of the foundational tests can help them to identify the most common sources of inflammation.

Testing for Food Sensitivities

Now is the time to decide whether you will run a food sensitivities test immediately or you'll wait until you have diversified your child's diet. To help you make the right decision, consider the following points:

- If your child's diet is very limited, it is probably not time to run a food sensitivity test (one exception is the MRT, discussed in Six).

- If your child eats a relatively diverse diet, but you suspect leaky gut, pathogens, or otherwise compromised health, running a food sensitivities test at the start of the health-building program is a good way to identify and remove problematic foods, and speed up the healing process.

- If you have diversified and expanded your child's diet for several months, running a food sensitivity panel may be useful to help you refine the diet and remove any potentially inflammatory foods.

- If many foods come back as reactive on a test and you remove them from the diet, you may want to re-run the test after several months to get the latest picture of what's causing reactions in your child's body (if anything). Likewise, after you re-introduce excluded foods you will probably want to run the test again after 3 to 6 months to ensure you catch inflammatory foods early and remove them from the diet.

- If you can't afford to run a quality food sensitivities test or there isn't one available in your area, I would recommend that you skip it for now.

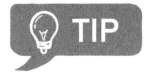

As an aside, because most food sensitivities tests require a blood draw, you may find that an at-home dried blood spot test is much more convenient and less stressful. The Great Plains Laboratory offers such a test, with the option to choose between the standard panel and one which includes a wider range of Asian foods (useful if your child's diet includes such foods). You will find a link to the test on the resources webpage for the book (along with any other similar tests I find in the future).

Hair Testing

The value for money a hair mineral analysis (HMA) provides cannot be overstated. When you get the HMA results, the following are of particular interest:

- Overall mineral levels
- Copper status
- Heavy metals being excreted

There are other more subtle insights we can glean from an HMA, such as the pattern of minerals and the ratios between some of them, but this is beyond the scope of this book. A skilled clinician will help you make sense of the finer points of the HMA.

Overall Mineral Levels

When analysing the mineral levels, your practitioner should pay attention to zinc, selenium, magnesium, and chromium. The levels of these in the hair track relatively closely with levels in the body. If any are low, it can signal a need to supplement extra. With autistic children, you will often find zinc, magnesium, and selenium to be low.

Copper Status

As we discussed in Chapter Four and Six, your child's zinc and copper status should be of particular interest to you, as they are often unbalanced in autistic children.

The copper level on the HMA may be elevated, normal, or low. When it is elevated on the first test, it most often indicates your child has a copper excess.

On the other hand, a low copper level often means there is an excess of copper where it shouldn't be - lodged in organs such as the liver.

You may notice that as you begin a protocol to balance the zinc and copper ratio (whether or not the initial copper was high or low), the next HMA results in an even higher copper level. This means the body has been eliminating copper and has dumped some in the hair in the process (remember that hair is an excretory tissue).

A later hair test is likely to show a lower copper level, which means the body has excreted the copper it wants to for now. Or, if the copper burden was especially high, you may see an even higher copper level, but eventually it should subside (though the body may repeat this process more than once if it senses it needs to). This is why re-testing every 3 to 4 months is recommended at the start of your child's program.

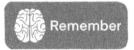

It's important to note that eliminating copper from the body can be an uncomfortable process, so you need to aware and prepared. I cover this in more detail later, in the section "Expecting Challenges".

Heavy Metals Being Excreted

Most often, a hair test will show some excretion of heavy metals. In my experience, mercury and aluminium are to be expected on any test result I review.

In fact, if heavy metals excretion is abnormally low, it is an indication that the person's detoxification capacities or overall health are diminished.

What you will usually find is that as you work to improve your child's health and wellbeing, subsequent HMA results will show higher excretion of toxic metals. Sometimes, you may be surprised to see significant elevations. This is a good thing, unless (in rare cases) there has been a strong acute exposure to metals from food or the environment. This is always a possibility (so make sure you rule it out), but more often than not it's the body using its newfound energy reserves to clean house.

What to Do About Pathogens

At this point, if you have run the OAT, a stool test, or both, you may have identified some pathogens that need to be eradicated.

Let's summarise the steps of supporting your child through the process of getting rid of the bad bugs and healing their gut:

- Implement a pathogen eradication protocol (herbals or antibiotics, and probiotics).
- Support the gut's healing (with a clean, non-inflammatory organic diet and supplements).
- Improve digestion (using digestive enzymes and by working to heal the gut).
- Remove foods to which your child has sensitivities.
- Remove other inflammatory factors such as environmental toxin exposures (heavy metals and chemicals).
- Allow time for healing and the protocol to work.
- Re-test to ensure pathogens are gone or to help you course-correct.
- Continue a healthy baseline diet, lifestyle, and supplementation program for your child.

As you can see, many of the recommendations throughout the *Autism Wellbeing Plan* promote gut healing and general gut health, directly and indirectly. That is why I keep saying that you need all the pieces of the puzzle in place to see the best results.

Let's look at some specifics about pathogen eradication that you need to know.

Antibiotics or Herbals?

Once you know what harmful critters have made a home for themselves in your child's gut, you may wonder what the best way is to get rid of them - antibiotics or herbal supplements.

Let's briefly cover some pros and cons of using each strategy, so you're aware of your options. Of course, you will follow your practitioner's advice, but it's good to be informed before you make a decision.

Pros and Cons of Antibiotics

Pros of antibiotics:

- They work quickly
- Simple and easy to take
- Sometimes, they may be the only or best option
- Can be lifesaving, especially with heavy infections

Cons of antibiotics:

- Antibiotics also kill our beneficial bacteria, thus disrupt the protective microbiota
- Many antibiotics only work on bacteria while leaving behind the yeast. The reduced beneficial bacteria in the gut leaves your child vulnerable to yeast overgrowths
- Some bacteria have become antibiotic resistant which means that treatment can kill good and bad bacteria, but leave behind the harmful opportunistic microbes such as *Clostridium difficile*[10] (and likely some yeast, ready to overgrow)
- There is evidence that oral antibiotics can suppress the excretion of mercury[11]
- May have other side effects

Pros and Cons of Herbals

Pros of herbal supplements:

- A gentler, more-natural way to balance the gut microbiota
- Less detrimental to the beneficial bacteria, in many cases
- May have "side-benefits", rather than side-effects, because many of the herbs have health-promoting qualities

Cons of herbal supplements:

- Because herbs tend to be gentler, benefits may take longer than antibiotics to take effect (herbal protocols can last anywhere from one to six months, whereas antibiotics are usually taken for up to a couple of weeks at a time)
- The herbal protocol may be more costly

Deciding Which Direction to Go

There are times when antibiotics are the best option to address gut infections, there is no doubt about it. Heavy or life-threatening infections need to be dealt with swiftly.

However, we have grossly over-used antibiotics in the past decades, and this has caused many bacteria to become resistant to a lot of them. It's wise to keep them as a last resort, if you can help it, because they can do as much harm as good when they disrupt the beneficial bacteria. This is especially amplified with kids whose microbiota and immune system may already be compromised. The initial infection may go away, but the negative effects will not be felt until weeks or months later.

Pathogen Eradication Protocols

Let's look at considerations around protocols to support pathogen eradication.

Probiotics

Probiotics should always be part of a pathogen eradication protocol. Not only are some probiotics anti-pathogenic in their own right, they also help to stabilise the microbiota and intestinal barrier. Some examples from scientific literature include:

- *Lactobacillus acidophilus GG* has been used successfully to control relapses of *Clostridium difficile* colitis.[12]
- *Lactobacillus acidophilus GG* was shown to reduce elevated levels of the *Clostridia* metabolite HPHPA (discussed in Chapter Three) in the urine of autistic study participants.[13]
- Certain *Bifidobacteria* and *Lactobacillus* strains produce a large amount of short-chain fatty acids, such as butyrate, that can inhibit *Candida albicans* growth.[14]
- *Lactobacillus acidophilus* has been shown to inhibit *Candida* growth. A reduction of a marker for *Candida* in the urine (D-arabinitol) also correlated with improved behaviours and ability to concentrate.[15]
- In an ASD study where they found microbiota imbalances and increased *Desulfovibrio*, a probiotic containing three strains of *Lactobacillus*, two strains of *Bifidobacteria*, and one strain of *Streptococcus* was able to decrease the levels of *Desulfovibrio* and improve the balance of the microbiota.[16]

Fungal Protocols

Below is a summary of the core yeast and mould protocols. Your practitioner may augment them based on your case and test results.

Basic Yeast Protocol

When yeast overgrowth such as *Candida* is detected, the basic protocol to address it would include:

- Herbal or prescription anti-fungal (e.g. Biocidin® or nystatin, respectively)
- Probiotics
- Low-sugar diet

The Mould Protocol

Addressing mould is similar to the yeast protocol, with some additional considerations.

The most crucial action is to reduce or eliminate the source of exposure, which is most often mould damage in your home or food contamination. Keep your child away from water damaged environments and avoid corn, peanuts, and other foods at risk of being contaminated.

A typical mould protocol may include:

- Anti-fungal medications or herbal supplements
- Probiotics
- Glutathione
- Binder supplements to absorb mycotoxins in the gut (e.g. zeolite, charcoal, NovaSil)
- Chlorophyllin
- Cholestyramine

Additionally, older children can use a sauna under your supervision to help with toxin elimination, if recommended by your health care provider.

Herbal Options

You can refer to Chapter Eleven for a list of herbs that you can use in your child's pathogen protocol.

I briefly mentioned Biocidin® in the previous chapter, but it's worth covering again because it is such a great product. (Again, I have no affiliation to any labs, tests, or other products. I just recommend quality stuff that works.)

Biocidin® is a herbal supplement that can be used to support pathogen eradication. It is a blend of various herbs that have anti-inflammatory, antioxidant, antimicrobial, anti-fungal, anti-biofilm, and other beneficial properties.

The advantage of Biocidin® is that it is available in liquid form that has a pleasant taste, which makes it easy to give to your child. You can use the dropper to drop it on their tongue or you can add the drops to water or juice.

Herbs in the Biocidin® mix include bilberry extract, noni, milk thistle, echinacea, goldenseal, garlic, black walnut, oregano oil, and others.

Prescription Antibiotics and Anti-Fungals

Your doctor will advise you on which antibiotics and anti-fungals to use, if you decide to go that route. I'll briefly cover a couple of commonly used ones.

Clostridium Difficile

Both vancomycin and metronidazole are two potential antibiotic options to address *Clostridium difficile*.[13][17] More recently, fidaxomicin has been shown to be effective in treating *Clostridium difficile* infections.

Vancomycin treatment has been shown to significantly, but temporarily, reduce autistic symptoms, with a gradual regression after treatment is stopped.[17] The regression may be because antibiotics can't kill the spores of some bacteria, which allows them to recolonise the gut. Vancomycin is minimally absorbed, which means that it remains in the gut and exerts most of its effects there, before being excreted in the stool.

Anti-Fungals

A popular anti-fungal, nystatin, can be used to address fungal infections such as *Candida* (though your clinician might have a better alternative, as many yeasts are now resistant to it). It's safe because it doesn't get absorbed, so it exerts its effects only in the gut.

Nystatin has been trialled on autistic children. The treatment was able to reduce the urine fungal markers on the organic acids test and overall the participants' CARS scores (an indicator for ASD severity) improved significantly. Simply put, the anti-fungal treatment helped to reduce autistic symptoms in the study group.[18]

Through my research, I've seen that some doctors use Diflucan (fluconazole), Sporanox (itraconazole), and Lamisil (terbinafine) as alternatives to nystatin, but there is no published research yet supporting their use for autistic children, just clinical experience. Those anti-fungals are absorbed into the body, so a much more cautious approach is warranted. Your doctor should be able to recommend the most effective option.

Die-Off Reactions During Pathogen Protocols

When pathogens are killed, they can release their toxins all at once. This can cause what is known as a "die-off" reaction (also known as a cleansing or Herxheimer reaction).

Some of the most common symptoms of a die-off reaction include:

- Nausea
- Fatigue
- Headache
- Irritability, moodiness
- Hyperactivity
- Sleep disturbances
- Rashes
- Itching
- Fever
- Self-stimulatory behaviour
- Digestive issues (bloating, discomfort, alternating diarrhoea and constipation)

In a severe die-off reaction, fever and lethargy may be accompanied by profuse sweating and heart palpitations.[13]

You need to be aware of the possibility of your child experiencing the reaction and not panic. It should typically last from three to seven days and may be quite variable. For instance, your child may be hyperactive at first, followed by a day or two of lethargy, before you see a noticeable improvement.[17]

If the reaction lasts longer than about seven days, it may be that your child is reacting to a supplement or something in the diet, or the protocol is too strong and your child is unable to cope with eliminating the die-off by-products. You never want your child to experience a severe reaction, of course, which is why gradually increasing the protocol is so important. This is easier to do with herbs than antibiotics.

Some ways you can mitigate the effects of the cleansing reaction include:

- Reducing the dosage of the pathogen protocol temporarily, depending on your practitioner's advice
- Using binder supplements like charcoal or zeolite to "mop-up" the die-off by-products in your child's gut so they don't get absorbed
- Keeping your child well-hydrated
- Feeding your child plenty of cooked vegetables and fibre to keep them pooping regularly

Charcoal can be somewhat constipating. If you ever need to use it, taking some magnesium citrate (away from the charcoal) can help to keep the stools moving.

Summaries: Improving Diet, Reducing Toxic Exposures, Sleep Hygiene, and Supplementation

Let's list the key takeaways around improving the diet, reducing toxic exposures, sleep hygiene, and supplementation.

Improving the Diet

Hopefully you've decided to at least give the gluten-free, casein-free (GFCF) diet a try. However, even if you think it's not yet time to try it, there are still many positive changes you can make to your child's diet. These include:

- Switching to organic whole foods
- Cooking more meals at home from scratch

- Reducing processed and junk foods
- Reducing additives and chemicals
- Diversifying the diet
- Emphasising chewing the food thoroughly
- Reinforcing mindful eating (switch off the TV or other screens during mealtimes)
- Avoiding drinking too much water right before, during, and one hour after meals (it dilutes digestive juices)

How to Record and Analyse Your Child's Food Intake

I know you're busy. But writing down what you feed your child for three to seven typical days is not difficult. If you follow the instructions below, you can quickly and easily see if the current diet covers your child's nutritional bases. You can also go to the resources webpage for this book to see a video of me creating an account and entering a day's worth of food data, followed by some quick analysis and some tips.

Basic steps to track your child's food intake:

- Go to https://cronometer.com/ and create a free account. Alternatively, download the free Cronometer app for Android or iPhone.
- When registering, enter your child's birth date (or thereabouts - you don't need to give the exact date if you wish), weight, and height.
- On the Diary page, add all the foods your child ate that day.
- If you've been keeping written food logs and want to enter them all at once, simply go back a few days in the calendar and input the data for several days. This will all make sense once you have the Cronometer app open or you watch my video.

When you've finished inputting the food data, take a closer look at the sections showing vitamins, minerals, lipids, and protein. There you want to scan for the following:

- Is intake of any vitamins or minerals very low?
- What is the ratio of omega-3 to omega-6 fatty acid intake?
- Is energy intake sufficient (and not too high)?

It's a good idea to hover over the individual nutrients to get an idea of which foods are providing them. See if you can spot any patterns.

For example, a day low in meat and high in plant foods is most likely a day low in zinc and high in copper. Take a look how much protein and fat your child eats in a typical day. Is intake of either of these crucial macronutrients very low? Kids' diets can very easily become carb-heavy, leaving them with few nutrients to build and repair their bodies (cells and tissues are mostly made from proteins and fats).

The insights you gain from this exercise will be worth the effort. You can even discuss your food logs with your practitioner to get advice and ideas on how you may enhance your child's diet.

Reducing Environmental Toxin Exposures

Remember the most salient points from Chapter Eight (and revisit it at times to refresh your memory, if you need):

- Get familiar with the Environmental Working Group's (EWG) online resources.
- Avoid plastic cooking utensils, storage boxes, and buying food in plastic containers. Avoid plastics with the recycling symbols 3, 6, and 7.
- Install affordable tap and shower filters.
- Use a HEPA air purifier to improve the air quality at home.
- Replace conventional cleaning products, soaps, shampoos, and other products with natural alternatives free from harsh chemicals.

Improving Sleep

Summary of improving your child's sleep hygiene and environment:

- Cool, quiet, and dark bedroom.
- Turn down bright lights one to two hours before sleep (using red LED bulbs reduces the impact on your family's sleep rhythms).
- Turn off screens *at least* one hour before bed, preferably more (and keep devices out of the bedroom).
- Reduce stimulating activities prior to bedtime.
- Have a consistent sleep schedule and routine, displayed prominently at home and adhered to strictly.
- Try not to switch the lights on in the middle of the night (consider red LEDs if you will need to).
- Avoid sugary or high-carbohydrate meals close to bedtime to

prevent blood-sugar fluctuations that may disturb sleep.

Supplementation

Remember the guidelines around supplementation:

- Introduce supplements one at a time.
- Go low and slow - begin with a small amount and gradually work up to the desired amount.
- Track your child's supplements in your journal (including your observations of their response to them).
- Quality and ingredients matter. Get your practitioner to help you, otherwise use the resources in this book and the free online course you get when you sign up to my mailing list.
- Supplements will never make up for a poor diet. Diet is the foundation of your house.

Supporting Toxin Elimination

You may be surprised to hear it, but the absolute best way to support toxin elimination is to get your child as healthy as possible. As soon as the body is given the raw materials and energy it needs, it will start pushing out the heavy metals and chemicals that have accumulated in its tissues.

We covered some supplements you can use to support your child's natural detoxification capacities in Chapter Eleven. We'll now briefly touch on two more methods that may be utilised in more serious cases of toxicity.

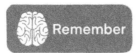

Remember

Of course, in all cases, you must remove as many sources of toxic exposure as possible, to prevent your child's detoxification systems from becoming overwhelmed.

Chelation Therapy

If your child's heavy metal burden is found to be extremely high, they may be a good candidate for chelation therapy.

Chelation therapy involves using special agents such as DMSA, DMPS, or EDTA to bind (chelate) the heavy metals circulating in your child's blood. The metals can then be safely excreted in the urine and poop.

It can be a life-saving procedure in cases of severe toxic burden, but it must always be performed by an experienced physician. Chelation carries with it certain risks, which you must be aware of before beginning this type of therapy. One of them is that the chelating agents used also bind with essential minerals such as zinc, iron, or selenium. The problem with this is that the circulating chelating agent "rips" those essential minerals indiscriminately out of enzymes, blood vessel walls, or other bodily tissues. This can destabilise the body.

Although experienced doctors know that they you need to supplement the person with minerals during chelation therapy, you need to be careful. Simply giving your child some minerals won't magically restore them in the places they were ripped from.

I've included links to further reading on the topic of heavy metal chelation on the resources webpage for the book.

Sauna

For older children whose test results show high levels of toxicity, sauna use under your supervision is an effective way to support detoxification. Virtually all kinds of toxins, from heavy metals to chemicals, can be excreted though sweat. Always get your health care provider's guidance before you decide to use a sauna.

Expecting Challenges

The journey to health is never linear. It's more like "two steps forward, one step back" much of the time, with some unexpected twists and turns, especially at the start of a health-building program.

This is because the body is incredibly complex. When one layer of dysfunction is addressed, it can take some time for it to adjust its biochemical processes to remain in balance (homeostasis).

Think about when you're spring cleaning your home. You don't magically have a clean house after you start. It's a dirty, messy activity with different jobs to get done. You don't take the trash out until the time is right, likewise you don't wipe the dust until the dirty work is finished.

It's the same with the healing process. The body needs nutrients and the removal of stressors, but it also needs time and rest to rebuild and repair.

I'll outline several common scenarios where your child may seem to get worse for a while. You need to be cognisant of these to avoid panicking needlessly if the situations arise. Of course, you always need to rule out acute toxic exposure or other medical emergencies first.

Some potential scenarios you can expect:

- **Die-off reactions** at the start of the pathogen eradication protocol. As I mentioned in an earlier section, keep your child well-hydrated and pooping regularly by providing them with plenty of fibre in the form of cooked vegetables. Magnesium citrate can be useful to keep the bowels moving. If the reaction is more severe, you may need to back off the pathogen protocol for some days. Keeping some charcoal or zeolite at home just in case is a good idea, as they can help absorb bacterial die-off in the gut and prevent it from getting into the bloodstream.

- **Dumping excess copper.** When there is an excess of biounavailable copper in the body, it can get stored in various organs such as the liver. As you work to balance your child's zinc and copper status, the body begins to excrete excess copper. Because it needs to get excreted through the blood, the blood copper temporarily becomes elevated, and may cause symptoms of copper excess such as anxiety, irritability, insomnia, nausea, digestive upset, and even skin breakouts. It's not a fun process, but the body needs to go through it on its way back to health, so you need to be prepared. Taking a hair sample at this time would usually show elevated copper levels - an indication that the body is getting rid of it through the various means it has to do so.

- **Excretion of high levels of toxic metals.** Similar to copper, when toxic metals are pushed out of the tissues in which they are lodged, they need to be transported out of the body. When the body gains vitality and has the right nutrients to do so, it starts the process. This can cause some temporary symptoms.

Taking a hair sample at this time often shows elevated mercury, aluminium, and occasionally other heavy metals, again indicating the body is excreting them.

- **Dumping of oxalates** when implementing the low oxalate diet due to elevated oxalic acid levels on the organic acids test. Oxalate crystals can lodge themselves in various tissues and organs in the body. When the influx of oxalate is reduced, the body can start dumping the stored oxalates. This can cause significant discomfort, which is why you need to lower dietary oxalates gradually. Refer to Chapter Four and Seven for a refresher on oxalates and the low oxalate diet, and Chapter Eleven for a list of supplements that can help with high oxalates.

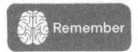

Please keep in mind that these reactions should be temporary and not overly severe. Always make sure you keep in close contact with your practitioner during challenging periods, and have them guide and advise you.

Monitoring Progress and Re-Testing

Let's look at some considerations around re-testing and course-correcting.

Remember that everything depends on your current resources and insurance coverage. Obviously, if you're well-covered or have the cash to spare, running tests more often will allow your practitioner to better fine-tune your child's protocol. That is within reason, of course. Please don't allow yourself to be suckered into excessive testing. That's not the answer. What is truly needed is the proper execution of the basics: organic and healthy diet, clean environment, proper supplementation, and solid sleep hygiene. Sure, testing will guide the process, but running ten tests won't do one iota of good for your child unless you do the fundamentals consistently well.

Guidelines on re-testing:

- **Organic acids test:** 3 to 6 months after first test, depending on initial findings. If many yeast and bacterial markers were elevated along with other imbalances (e.g. elevated oxalate, nutrient or glutathione deficiencies, indicators for mitochondrial dysfunction), then re-test sooner to ensure the program is addressing said imbalances. If the OAT only shows some elevated yeast and bacteria, and you use a standard herbal protocol (e.g. Biocidin® and probiotics), you can wait a bit longer for the re-test to see if the protocol was effective. Once you have restored a good baseline level of health in your child, you may want to run the test once or twice a year to keep an eye on yeast or bacterial overgrowths, or other imbalances. The earlier you catch them, the better.
- **Stool test:** at least 30 days after finishing a pathogen eradication protocol. You want to allow time for the gut microbiota to stabilise so you can see whether the infection has been permanently ousted (testing during a protocol may show no infection or overgrowth, but the bugs may return after the herbs or antibiotics are stopped).
- **Blood tests:** apart from the regular check-ups your doctor runs, you will want to monitor any markers that were found to be out of balance at the start.
- **Hair mineral analysis:** as explained earlier, running these every 3-4 months is an affordable way to monitor your child's mineral balance and toxic metal excretion, as well as more subtle mineral patterns and ratios.

Remember to record the important details in your journal for quick reference. It's easy to forget little things that happen on a day-to-day basis with our frantic fast-paced lifestyles. Having your observations written down will allow you to periodically review them and get new insights into what is working well for your child. You may even be surprised how much progress your youngster has made in several months in terms of their overall health.

Example Protocol and Sequence: The First 3 to 6 Months

Here is a typical scenario and a standard health-building protocol. I will keep it simple, but it should give you a clear example of how to go about structuring a health-building program for your child.

<u>Scenario:</u>

Four-year-old child with a self-limited diet that is heavy in wheat and milk products, and some sweets. The child avoids meat and vegetables but eats the occasional fruit. They are often constipated, and their sleep is not great (night-time awakenings and occasional drowsiness in the morning).

<u>Testing:</u>

The parents decide to run the following tests at the start:

- Organic acids test (OAT)
- Hair mineral analysis (HMA)
- Basic blood work

Their practitioner recommends against running the food sensitivities test at this time as it is unlikely to provide much clinical value (due to the limited diet). The parents decide to run a stool pathogen test in a few months to conserve resources.

<u>Initial protocol (first month):</u>

While waiting for the OAT and HMA results, the parents order the core five supplements. Because their child is constipated often, they begin the supplements in the following order: probiotics, digestive enzymes, cod liver oil, multivitamin, and finally the calcium and magnesium. This process takes three weeks.

The practitioner suggests using melatonin as a short-term measure to support more restorative sleep, while any underlying contributors to poor sleep are identified and addressed.

The parents begin swapping in gluten-free products for wheat-based ones and gradually begin reducing milk products. Having learnt about the EWG's Dirty Dozen and Clean Fifteen list (discussed in Chapter

Eight), they start buying organic tomatoes, potatoes, and apples to re-duce some potential pesticide residues.

Other actions the parents decide to take:

- Order an inexpensive faucet filter to improve the water quality for the whole family
- Replace soaps with safer alternatives from the health store
- Stop using the fabric softener and buy washing powder from the health store after the current box is finished
- Start dimming the lights as sleep time approaches
- Turn off all screens at least one hour before bed

Test results:

Blood test results arrive within the first week of testing with the fol-lowing findings:

- Zinc is trending toward the bottom of the reference range
- Copper is close to the top of the range
- Vitamin D is on the low side, but not deficient
- Homocysteine is slightly elevated (a marker for inflammation)

It takes 3-4 weeks for the OAT and HMA results to arrive. The organic acids test indicates:

- *Candida overgrowth*
- *Clostridium difficile presence*
- Elevated oxalates
- Low-normal vitamin B6 level

The hair mineral analysis indicates:

- Elevated copper
- Low zinc, magnesium, and selenium
- Moderate aluminium and mercury levels

Protocol after lab tests:

The sequence of supplements after the blood tests:

- Zinc

- Vitamin B_6, methylfolate, and B_{12} complex liquid
- TMG powder
- (Note that vitamin D wasn't added to the protocol as the multivitamin supplement contains it, the practitioner decides to re-evaluate after the next blood test)

Protocol additions after the OAT and HMA results arrive:

- Biocidin® (one drop per 5kg (10 lbs) of bodyweight, starting with one drop and gradually increasing it)
- Saccharomyces boulardii probiotic in addition to current probiotic
- Extra selenium

Due to the elevated oxalates, the parents begin reducing food high in oxalates slowly, replacing them with lower oxalate substitutes.

Other supplements the practitioner recommends for general support:

- Carnitine
- Taurine in the evening
- Small amount of glycine and NAC to support glutathione production

Re-tests:

After 3-4 months, the parents have the option to re-test with the OAT or run a stool pathogen screening. They don't have insurance cover, so they decide to wait another two months before re-testing with the OAT. In the meantime, they have managed to get a free stool pathogen screening from their local clinic. The practitioner uses this to evaluate how the pathogen protocol is working and to detect potential parasites and bacteria not specifically tested for by the OAT.

After 3-4 months, the next hair test shows elevated copper and higher amounts of mercury and aluminium, indicating that their child is eliminating them. Overall, a good sign.

Next steps:

At this point, the parents are motivated by the positive progress they see in their child's health. They continue the baseline healthy diet and seek out ways to incrementally improve it. While setbacks do happen, they do their best to bounce back from them. They understand that perfection is not the goal, rather doing the basics consistently is the most important thing. Shopping for food and cooking gluten-free meals is now much easier.

I hope this gives you a solid understanding of how a health-building program is designed and implemented. You can use this template to create one for your child, with the help of your practitioner.

Wrap-up

In this final chapter of the *Autism Wellbeing Plan*, we consolidated everything you learnt in the book into a cohesive plan to:

- Track your child's health journey in your journal.
- Rule out or identify potentially serious disorders as soon as possible.
- Identify the most common imbalances using the foundational lab tests.
- Understand when to pursue more advanced testing.
- Design suitable pathogen eradication protocols to address gut infections.
- Improve your child's diet, reduce toxic exposures, establish positive habits to promote restorative sleep, and supplement vital nutrients.
- Monitor and re-test to ensure the program is addressing the identified imbalances.
- Anticipate challenges along the way and course correct as needed.

Before you go ahead and implement your child's health-building program, please turn the page to see how I can continue to support you on your journey.

CLOSING THOUGHTS

Thank you for investing the time to read the *Autism Wellbeing Plan*. I sincerely hope that you use the information in here to greatly improve your child's wellbeing, and by extension, your whole family's quality of life. I poured my heart and soul into this book because I honestly believe the current system has failed you miserably, and you deserve much more support than you're receiving. My hope is that books like this and the continued work of the researchers and clinicians pushing us in the right direction will help more children around the world live healthier, happier lives.

As a reminder, you'll find many more resources here: **https://christianyordanov.com/autism-wellbeing-plan-resources/** Don't forget to subscribe to my mailing list to get access to the free video course on choosing quality supplements for your child, and to receive future articles, videos, research, and other content you may find useful or interesting.

Please send me an email (cy@christianyordanov.com) with your questions and feedback about the book. As I mentioned at the outset, if your feedback, comments, or questions help me improve the *Autism Wellbeing Plan*, I'll send you a complimentary paperback of the next edition (with an acknowledgement in the book, if you're happy with that).

Lastly, if you found this information useful, please share the book with others that may find it helpful. Also, please take a couple of minutes to leave an honest review on Amazon, I would be eternally grateful. You've no idea how crucial reviews are to spread the message to more parents that may benefit from it. Thank you!

I wish you all the very best on your journey!

Christian Yordanov

ABOUT THE AUTHOR

Christian Yordanov is a Certified Functional Diagnostic Nutrition® Practitioner, health researcher, educator and coach. His main areas of research are autism spectrum disorders, children's health, preparing for a healthy pregnancy, and longevity.

Website: https://christianyordanov.com/

Podcast: https://autismwellbeingplan.buzzsprout.com/ (Search for "Autism Wellbeing Plan" in your favourite podcast player.)

ACKNOWLEDGEMENTS

To my amazing partner, Ingrida, thank you for your limitless support, encouragement, and help along this journey. Thank you for enduring my incessant talking about this project and my complaining about how arduous it was to research and produce a book! I love you.

To my dear friend Kathleen Dixon, from Breather Better OC, thank you for your invaluable input on this book. You've no idea how much you helped me!

To Patrick McKeown, from the Buteyko Clinic, thank you for your time in reviewing and contributing to the section on breathing.

To all my mentors and colleagues from the Association of Functional Diagnostic Nutrition® Practitioners, thank you for continuing to push the envelope and expand our positive impact on the world. Big shout out to Reed Davis, Brandon Molle, and Brendan Vermeire - you guys are awesome!

Last, but certainly not least, my most sincere gratitude goes out to the many researchers and clinicians whose shoulders I stand on. You are the real heroes. I applaud you for your contributions to this incredibly important field.

REFERENCES

Introduction

1. Adams JB, Johansen LJ, Powell LD, Quig D, Rubin RA (2011) Gastrointes-
    tinal flora and gastrointestinal status in children with autism comparisons
    to typical children and correlation with autism severity. BMC Gastroen-
    terol 11:22.
2. Finegold SM, Downes J, Summanen PH. Microbiology of regressive au-
    tism. Anaerobe 2012;18:2602.
3. Altieri L, Neri C, Sacco R, Curatolo P, Benvenuto A, Muratori F, et al.
    Urinary p-cresol is elevated in small children with severe autism spectrum
    disorder. Biomarkers (2011) 16:25260. doi:10.3109/1354750X.2010.548010.
4. Gabriele S, Sacco R, Altieri L, Neri C, Urbani A, Bravaccio C, Riccio MP,
    Iovene MR, Bombace F, deMagistris L, Persico AM. Slow intestinal transit
    contributes to elevate urinary p-cresol level in Italian autistic children. Au-
    tism Res. 2015;. doi:10.1002/aur.1571.
5. Nikolov RN, Bearss KE, Lettinga J, et al. (2009) Gastrointestinal symp-
    toms in a sample of children with pervasive developmental disorders. Jour-
    nal of Autism and Developmental Disorders 39(3): 405-413.
6. Chaidez, Virginia & Hansen, Robin & Hertz-Picciotto, Irva. (2013). Gas-
    trointestinal Problems in Children with Autism, Developmental Delays or
    Typical Development. Journal of autism and developmental disorders. 44.
    10.1007/s10803-013-1973-x.
7. Adams, J.B.; Audhya, T.; McDonough-Means, S.; Rubin, R.A.; Quig, D.;
    Geis, E.; Gehn, E.; Loresto, M.; Mitchell, J.; Atwood, S.; et al. Nutritional
    and Metabolic Status of Children with Autism vs. Neurotypical Children,
    and the Association with Autism Severity. Nutr. Metab. 2011, 8, 34.
8. Mostafa GA, El-Gamal HA, El-Wakkad ASE, El-Shorbagy OE, Hamza
    MM. Polyunsaturated fatty acids, carnitine and lactate as biological mark-
    ers of brain energy in autistic children. Int J Child Neuropsychiatry 2005; 2:
    179-188.
9. Li, Si-Ou & Wang, Jia-Liang & Bjorklund, Geir & Zhao, Wei-Na & Yin,
    Chang-Hao. (2014). Serum copper and zinc levels in individuals with au-
    tism spectrum disorders. Neuroreport. 25. 10.1097/WNR.0000000000000251.
10. Priya MD, Geetha A Level of Trace Elements (Copper, Zinc, Magnesium
    and Selenium) and Toxic Elements (Lead and Mercury) in the Hair and
    Nail of Children with Autism. Biol Trace Ele Res 2010:1-11

11. Russo AJ, Bazin AP, Bigega R, Carlson RS 3rd, Cole MG, Contreras DC, et al. Plasma copper and zinc concentration in individuals with autism correlate with selected symptom severity. Nutr Metab Insights 2012; 5:41-47.

12. Elsheshtawy, E., Tobar, S., Sherra, K., Atallah, S., Elkasaby, R., 2011. Study of some biomarkers in hair of children with autism. Middle East Curr. Psychiatry 18 (1), 6-10.

13. Blaurock-Busch E, Amin OR, Dessoki HH, Rabah T. Toxic Metals and Essential Elements in Hair and Severity of Symptoms among Children with Autism. Maedica (Buchar) 2012;7(1):38-48.

14. Ashwood, P., Krakowiak, P., Hertz-Picciotto, I., Hansen, R., Pessah, I., and Van De Water, J. (2011). Elevated plasma cytokines in autism spectrum disorders provide evidence of immune dysfunction and are associated with impaired behavioral outcome. Brain Behav. Immun. 25, 40-45. doi: 10.1016/j.bbi.2010.08.003.

15. Goyal, Daniel & Miyan, Jaleel. (2014). Neuro-Immune Abnormalities in Autism and Their Relationship with the Environment: A Variable Insult Model for Autism. Frontiers in endocrinology. 5. 29. 10.3389/fendo.2014.00029.

16. Onore C, Careaga M, Ashwood P. The role of immune dysfunction in the pathophysiology of autism. Brain Behav Immun (2012) 26(3):383-92. doi:10.1016/j.bbi.2011.08.007

17. Ashwood P, Enstrom A, Krakowiak P, Hertz-Picciotto I, Hansen RL, Croen LA, et al. Decreased transforming growth factor beta1 in autism: a potential link between immune dysregulation and impairment in clinical behavioral outcomes. J Neuroimmunol (2008) 204(12):149-53. doi:10.1016/j.jneuroim.2008. 07.006.

18. Adams, J.B., Baral, M., Geis, E., Mitchell, J., Ingram, J., Hensley, A., et al., 2009. The severity of autism is associated with toxic metal body burden and red blood cell glutathione levels. J. Toxicol. 2009, 532640.

19. Geier, D.A., Kern, J.K., King, P.G., Sykes, L.K., Geier, M.R., 2012. Hair toxic metal concentrations and autism spectrum disorder severity in young children. Int. J. Environ. Res. Public Health 9 (12), 4486-4497.

20. Blaurock-Busch, E., Amin, O.R., Dessoki, H.H., Rabah, T., 2012. Toxic metals and essential elements in hair and severity of symptoms among children with autism. Maedica 7 (1), 38-48.

21. Adams, J.B., Audhya, T., McDonough-Means, S., Rubin, R.A., Quig, D., Geis, E., et al., 2013. Toxicological status of children with autism vs. neurotypical children and the association with autism severity. Biol. Trace Elem. Res. 151 (2), 171-180.

22. Boggess, Andrew & Faber, Scott & Kern II, John & Kingston, H. M. Skip. (2016). Mean serum-level of common organic pollutants is predictive of behavioral severity in children with autism spectrum disorders. Scientific reports. 6. 26185. 10.1038/srep26185.

23. Mannion, A., Leader, G., & Healy, O. (2013). An investigation of comorbid psychological disorders, sleep problems, gastrointestinal symptoms and epilepsy in children and adolescents with autism spectrum disorder. Research in Autism Spectrum Disorders, 7(1), 35-42.

24. Simonoff, E., Pickles, A., Charman, T., Chandler, S., Loucas, T., & Baird, G. (2008). Psychiatric disorders in children with autism spectrum disorders: Prevalence, comorbidity and associated factors in a population-driven sample. Journal of the American Academy Child and Adolescent Psychiatry, 47(8), 921-929 http://dx.doi.org/10.1097/CHI.0b013e318179964f.

25. Leyfer, O. T., Folstein, S. E., Bacalman, S., Davis, N. O., Dinh, E., Morgan, J., et al. (2006). Comorbid psychiatric disorders in children with autism: Interview development and rates of disorders. Journal of Autism and Developmental Disorders, 36, 849–861. http://dx.doi.org/10.1007/s10803-006-0123-0.

26. Morris, Zoë & Wooding, Steven & Grant, Jonathan. (2011). The answer is 17 years, what is the question: Understanding time lags in translational research. Journal of the Royal Society of Medicine. 104. 510-20. 10.1258/jrsm.2011.110180.

Chapter One

1. Dinan, T. G., Stilling, R. M., Stanton, C., and Cryan, J. F. (2015). Collective unconscious: how gut microbes shape human behavior. J. Psychiatr. Res. 63, 1-9. doi: 10.1016/j.jpsychires.2015.02.021.

2. Bermon S, Petriz B, Kajeniene A, Prestes J, Castell L, Franco OL (2015) The microbiota: an exercise immunology perspective. Exerc Immunol Rev 21:70-79.

3. Nicholson JK, Holmes E, Kinross J, et al. Host-gut microbiota metabolic interactions. Science. 2012;336(6086):1262–7.

4. Guzman JR, Conlin VS, Jobin C. Diet, microbiome, and the intestinal epithelium: an essential triumvirate? Biomed Res Int. 2013; 2013:425146.

5. Buie, T. (2015). Potential Etiologic Factors of Microbiome Disruption in Autism. Clinical Therapeutics, 37(5), 976–983. doi:10.1016/j.clinthera.2015.04.001

6. Wu, H. J., and Wu, E. (2012). The role of gut microbiota in immune homeostasis and autoimmunity. Gut Microbes 3, 414. doi: 10.4161/gmic.19320.

7. Claus SP, Ellero SL, Berger B, et al. Colonization-induced host-gut microbial metabolic interaction. MBio. 2011;2(2):e271-e210.

8. Shenderov BA, Midtvedt T. Epigenomic programing: a future way to health? Microb Ecol Health Dis. 2014;25:24145.

9. Alenghat T. Epigenomics and the microbiota. Toxicol Pathol. 2015;43(1):101–6.

10. Diaz Heijtz R, Wang S, Anuar F, et al. Normal gut microbiota modulates brain development and behavior. Proc Natl Acad Sci U S A. 2011;108(7):3047–52.

11. Coury DL, Ashwood P, Fasano A, et al. Gastrointestinal conditions in children with autism spectrum disorder: developing a research agenda. Pediatrics. 2012;130(Suppl 2):S160-S168.

12. Fond G, Boukouaci W, Chevalier G, Regnault A, Eberl G, Hamdani N, et al. The psychomicrobiotic: targeting microbiota in major psychiatric disorders: a systematic review. Pathol Biol. (2015) 63:35–42. doi: 10.1016/j.patbio.2014.10.003.

13. Cristiano, C., Lama, A., Lembo, F., Mollica, M. P., Calignano, A., & Mattace Raso, G. (2018). Interplay Between Peripheral and Central Inflammation in Autism Spectrum Disorders: Possible Nutritional and Therapeutic Strategies. Frontiers in Physiology, 9. doi:10.3389/fphys.2018.00184.

14. Li, Qian & Zhou, Jun-Mei. (2016). The microbiota-gut-brain axis and its potential therapeutic role in autism spectrum disorder. Neuroscience. 324. 10.1016/j.neuroscience.2016.03.013.

15. Stilling, Roman & Dinan, Timothy & Cryan, John. (2013). Microbial Genes, Brain & Behaviour - Epigenetic Regulation of the Gut-Brain Axis.. Genes, brain, and behavior. 13. 10.1111/gbb.12109.

16. Kraneveld, Aletta & De Theije, Caroline & Heesch, Floor & Borre, Yuliya & Kivit, Sander & Olivier, Berend & Korte, S. Mechiel & Garssen, J.. (2013). The Neuro-Immune Axis: Prospect for Novel Treatments of Mental Disorders.. Basic & clinical pharmacology & toxicology. 114. 10.1111/bcpt.12154.

17. Mayer, Emeran. (2011). Gut feelings: The emerging biology of gut-brain communication. Nature reviews. Neuroscience. 12. 453-66. 10.1038/nrn3071.

18. Williams BL, Hornig M, Buie T, et al. Impaired carbohydrate digestion and transport and mucosal dysbiosis in the intestines of children with autism and gastrointestinal disturbances. PLoS One. 2011;6(9):e24585.

19. Wang L, Christophersen CT, Sorich MJ, Gerber JP, Angley MT, Conlon MA. Increased abundance of Sutterella spp. and Ruminococcus torques in feces of children with autism spectrum disorder. Mol Autism. 2013;4(1):42.

20. Wang L, Conlon MA, Christophersen CT, Sorich MJ, Angley MT. Gastrointestinal microbiota and metabolite biomarkers in children with autism spectrum disorders. Biomark Med. 2014;8(3):331–44.

21. Kang DW, Park JG, Ilhan ZE, et al. Reduced incidence of Prevotella and other fermenters in intestinal microflora of autistic children. PLoS One. 2013;8(7):e68322.

22. Krajmalnik-Brown R, Lozupone C, Kang DW, Adams JB. Gut bacteria in children with autism spectrum disorders: challenges and promise of studying how a complex community influences a complex disease. Microb Ecol Health Dis. 2015;26:26914.

23. Bilbo SD, Nevison CD, Parker W. A model for the induction of autism in the ecosystem of the human body: the anatomy of a modern pandemic? Microb Ecol Health Dis. 2015;26:26253.

24. Montgomery RK, Mulberg AE, Grand RJ. Development of the human gastrointestinal tract: Twenty years of progress. Gastroenterology (1999) 116:702-31. doi: 10.1016/S0016-5085(99)70193-9.

25. Buie T, Fuchs GJ, Furuta GT, Kooros K, Levy J, Lewis JD, Wershil BK, Winter H: Recommendations for evaluation and treatment of common gastrointestinal problems in children with ASDs. Pediatrics 2010, 125(Suppl 1):S19-29.

26. Nikolov, R. N., Bearss, K. E., Lettinga, J., Erickson, C., Rodowski, M., Aman, M. G., et al. (2009). Gastrointestinal symptoms in a sample of children with pervasive developmental disorders. Journal of Autism and Developmental Disorders, 30, 405–413 http://dx.doi.org/10.1007/s10803-008-0637-8.

27. Adams JB, Johansen LJ, Powell LD, Quig D, Rubin RA (2011) Gastrointestinal flora and gastrointestinal status in children with autism comparisons to typical children and correlation with autism severity. BMC Gastroenterol 11:22.

28. Chaidez, Virginia & Hansen, Robin & Hertz-Picciotto, Irva. (2013). Gastrointestinal Problems in Children with Autism, Developmental Delays or Typical Development. Journal of autism and developmental disorders. 44. 10.1007/s10803-013-1973-x.

29. Sandler RH, Finegold SM, Bolte ER, Buchanan CP, Maxwell AP, Väisänen ML, Nelson MN, Wexler HM: Short-term benefit from oral vancomycin treatment of regressive-onset autism. Journal of Child Neurology 2000, 15(7):429-435.

30. Melmed R, Schneider C, Fabes R, Philips J, Reichelt K. Metabolic markers and gastrointestinal symptoms in children with autism and related disorders. J Pediatr Gastroenterol Nutr. (2000) 31(Suppl. 2):S31.

31. Valicenti-McDermott M, McVicar K, Rapin I, Wershil BK, Cohen H, Shinnar S. Frequency of gastrointestinal symptoms in children with autistic spectrum disorders and association with family history of autoimmune disease. J Dev Behav Pediatr. (2006) 27(Suppl. 2):S12836. doi: 10.1097/00004703-200604002-00011.

32. Buie T, Campbell DB, Fuchs, G. J. I. I. I., Furuta GT, Levy J, Vandewater J, et al. Evaluation, diagnosis, and treatment of gastrointestinal disorders in individuals with ASDs: a consensus report. Pediatrics (2010) 125(Suppl.1):S118. doi:10.1542/peds.2009-1878C.

33. Wang L, Christophersen CT, Sorich MJ, Gerber JP, Angley MT, Conlon MA. Low relative abundances of the mucolytic bacterium Akkermansia muciniphila and Bifidobacterium spp. in feces of children with autism. Appl Environ Microbiol. (2011) 77:671821. doi:10.1128/AEM.05212-11.

34. Carr, Edward & Owen-DeSchryver, Jamie. (2007). Physical Illness, Pain, and Problem Behavior in Minimally Verbal People with Developmental Disabilities. Journal of autism and developmental disorders. 37. 413-24. 10.1007/s10803-006-0176-0.

35. McAtee M, Carr EG, Schulte C, et al. (2004) A contextual assessment inventory for problem behavior: initial development. Journal of Positive Behavior Interventions 6(3):148-165.

36. Mazurek MO, Vasa RA, Kalb LG, Kanne SM, Rosenberg D, Keefer A, Murray DS, Freedman B, Lowery LA (2013) Anxiety, sensory over-responsivity, and gastrointestinal problems in children with autism spectrum disorders. J Abnorm Child Psychol 41:165-176.

37. Nikolov RN, Bearss KE, Lettinga J, et al. (2009) Gastrointestinal symptoms in a sample of children with pervasive developmental disorders. Journal of Autism and Developmental Disorders 39(3): 405-413.

38. Maenner MJ, Arneson CL, Levy SE, et al. (2012) Brief report: association between behavioral features and gastrointestinal problems in children with autism spectrum disorder. Journal of Autism Spectrum Disorders 42: 1520--1525.

39. Vojdani A. Food immune reactivity and neuroautoimmunity. Funct Neurol Rehabil Ergon, 2014; 4(2-3):175-195.

40. Fasano A. Physiological, pathological, and therapeutic implications of zonulin-mediated intestinal barrier modulation: living life on the edge of the wall. Am J Pathol. 2008;173(5):1243-1252.

41. Tripathi A, Lammers KM, Goldblum S, et al. Identification of human zonulin, a physiological modulator of tight junctions, as prehaptoglobin-2. Proc Natl Acad Sci USA. 2009;106(39):16799-16804

42. Lerner A, Matthias T. Changes in intestinal tight junction permeability associated with industrial food additives explain the rising incidence of autoimmune disease. Autoimmun Rev, 2015; 14(6):479-489. doi: 10.1016/j.autrev.2015.01.009.

43. de Magistris L, Familiari V, Pascotto A, Sapone A, Frolli A, Iardino P, et al. Alterations of the intestinal barrier in patients with autism spectrum disorders and in their first-degree relatives. J Pediatr Gastroenterol Nutr. (2010) 51:418–24. doi: 10.1097/MPG.0b013e3181dcc4a5.

44. Horvath K, Perman JA. Autism and gastrointestinal symptoms. Curr Gastroenterol Rep. 2002;4(3):251-258.

45. D'Eufemia P, Celli M, Finocchiaro R, et al. Abnormal intestinal permeability in children with autism. Acta Paediatr. 1996;85(9):1076-1079.

46. deMagistris L, Picardi A, Siniscalco D, Riccio MP, Sapone A, Cariello R, Abbadessa S, Medici N, Lammers KM, Schiraldi C, Iardino P, Marotta R, Tolone C, Fasano A, Pascotto A, Bravaccio C. Antibodies against food antigens in patients with autistic spectrum disorders (ASDs). Biomed Res Int. 2013;. doi:10.1155/2013/729349.

47. Iovene MR, Bombace F, Maresca R, Sapone A, Iardino P, Picardi A, et al. Intestinal Dysbiosis and Yeast Isolation in Stool of Subjects with Autism Spectrum Disorders. Mycopathologia. 2016.

48. Adams, J.B.; Audhya, T.; McDonough-Means, S.; Rubin, R.A.; Quig, D.; Geis, E.; Gehn, E.; Loresto, M.; Mitchell, J.; Atwood, S.; et al. Nutritional and Metabolic Status of Children with Autism vs. Neurotypical Children, and the Association with Autism Severity. Nutr. Metab. 2011, 8, 34.

49. Ghanizadeh, Ahmad & Akhondzadeh, Shahin & Hormozi, M & Makarem, Ali & Abotorabi-Zarchi, M & Firoozabadi, Ali. (2012). Glutathione-Related Factors and Oxidative Stress in Autism, A Review. Current medicinal chemistry. 19. 4000-5. 10.2174/092986712802002572.

50. Rose S, Melnyk S, Pavliv O, et al. Evidence of oxidative damage and inflammation associated with low glutathione redox status in the autism brain. Transl Psychiatry. 2012;2:e134.

51. Rossignol DA, Frye RE. Evidence linking oxidative stress, mitochondrial dysfunction, and inflammation in the brain of individuals with autism. Front Physiol. 2014;5:150.

52. Melnyk S, Fuchs GJ, Schulz E, et al. Metabolic imbalance associated with methylation dysregulation and oxidative damage in children with autism. J Autism Dev Disord. 2012;42(3):367–77.

53. Frye RE, Delatorre R, Taylor H, et al. Redox metabolism abnormalities in autistic children associated with mitochondrial disease. Transl Psychiatry. 2013;3:e273.

54. Geier DA, Kern JK, Garver CR, Adams JB, Audhya T, Geier MR: A prospective study of transsulfuration biomarkers in autistic disorders. Neurochem Res 2009, 34(2):386-93, Erratum in: Neurochem Res. 2009, 34(2):394.

55. James SJ, Cutler P, Melnyk S, Jernigan S, Janak L, Gaylor DW, Neubrander JA: Metabolic biomarkers of increased oxidative stress and impaired methylation capacity in children with autism. Am J Clin Nutr 2004, 80(6):1611-7.

56. James SJ, Melnyk S, Jernigan S, Cleves MA, Halsted CH, Wong DH, Cutler P, Bock K, Boris M, Bradstreet JJ, Baker SM, Gaylor DW: Metabolic endophenotype and related genotypes are associated with oxidative stress in children with autism. Am J Med Genet B Neuropsychiatr Genet 2006, 141:947-956.

57. James SJ, Melnyk S, Fuchs G, Reid T, Jernigan S, Pavliv O, Hubanks A, Gaylor DW: Efficacy of methylcobalamin and folinic acid treatment on glutathione redox status in children with autism. Am J Clin Nutr 2009,89(1):425-30.

58. Ghezzo, A.; Visconti, P.; Abruzzo, P.M.; Bolotta, A.; Ferreri, C.; Gobbi, G.; Malisardi, G.; Manfredini, S.; Marini, M.; Nanetti, L.; et al. Oxidative stress and erythrocyte membrane alterations in children with autism: Correlation with clinical features. PLoS ONE 2013, 8, e66418.

59. Al-Gadani, Y., El-Ansary, A., Attas, O., Al-Ayadhi, L., 2009. Metabolic biomarkersrelated to oxidative stress and antioxidant status in Saudi autistic children.Clin. Biochem. 42, 1032–1040.

60. Al-Yafee, Y.A., Al-Ayadhi, L.Y., Haq, S.H., El-Ansary, A.K., 2011. Novel metabolicbiomarkers related to sulfur-dependent detoxification pathways in autistic patients of Saudi Arabia. BMC Neurol. 11, 139.

61. Han, Y., Xi, Q.Q., Dai, W., Yang, S.H., Gao, L., Su, Y.Y., et al., 2015. Abnormal transsulfuration metabolism and reduced antioxidant capacity in Chinese children with autism spectrum disorders. Int. J. Dev. Neurosci. 46, 27–32.

62. Paşca, S.P., Dronca, E., Kaucsár, T., Craciun, E.C., Endreffy, E., Ferencz, B.K., et al.,2009. One carbon metabolism disturbances and the C677T MTHFR genepolymprhism in children with autism spectrum disorders. J. Cell Mol. Med. 13,4229–4238.

63. Adams, James & Audhya, Tapan & McDonough-Means, Sharon & Rubin, Robert & Quig, David & Geis, Elizabeth & Gehn, Eva & Loresto, Melissa & Mitchell, Jessica & Atwood, Sharon & Barnhouse, Suzanne & Lee, Wondra. (2011). Effect of a vitamin/mineral supplement on children and adults with autism. BMC pediatrics. 11. 111. 10.1186/1471-2431-11-111.

64. Daneman, R., & Prat, A. (2015). The Blood–Brain Barrier. Cold Spring Harbor Perspectives in Biology, 7(1), a020412. doi:10.1101/cshperspect.a020412.

65. Adinolfi M. The development of the human blood-CSF-brain barrier. Dev Med Child Neurol 1985; 27: 532-37.

Chapter Two

1. Hughes, Heather & Mills Ko, Emily & Rose, Destanie & Ashwood, Paul. (2018). Immune Dysfunction and Autoimmunity as Pathological Mechanisms in Autism Spectrum Disorders. Frontiers in Cellular Neuroscience. 12. 10.3389/fncel.2018.00405.

2. Goyal, Daniel & Miyan, Jaleel. (2014). Neuro-Immune Abnormalities in Autism and Their Relationship with the Environment: A Variable Insult Model for Autism. Frontiers in endocrinology. 5. 29. 10.3389/fendo.2014.00029.

3. Cohly, H.H.; Panja, A. Immunological findings in autism. Int. Rev. Neurobiol., 2005, 71, 317-41.

4. Ashwood, P.; Wakefield, A.J. Immune activation of peripheral blood and mucosal CD3+ lymphocyte cytokine profiles in children with autism and gastrointestinal symptoms. J. Neuroimmunol., 2006, 173, 126-34.

5. Ashwood, P.; Wills, S.; Van de Water, J. The immune response in autism: a new frontier for autism research. J. Leukoc. Biol., 2006, 80, 1-15.

6. Vojdani, Aristo & Lambert, Jama & Vojdani, Elroy. (2017). Blood-based markers in autism spectrum disorders Blood-based markers in autism spectrum disorders. Internal Medicine. 3.

7. Onore C, Careaga M, Ashwood P. The role of immune dysfunction in the pathophysiology of autism. Brain Behav Immun (2012) 26(3):383-92. doi:10.1016/j.bbi.2011.08.007.

8. Ashwood, P., Krakowiak, P., Hertz-Picciotto, I., Hansen, R., Pessah, I., and Van De Water, J. (2011). Elevated plasma cytokines in autism spectrum disorders provide evidence of immune dysfunction and are associated with impaired behavioral outcome. Brain Behav. Immun. 25, 40-45. doi: 10.1016/j.bbi.2010.08.003

9. Ashwood P, Enstrom A, Krakowiak P, Hertz-Picciotto I, Hansen RL, Croen LA, et al. Decreased transforming growth factor beta1 in autism: a potential link between immune dysregulation and impairment in clinical behavioral outcomes. J Neuroimmunol (2008) 204(12):149-53. doi:10.1016/j.jneuroim.2008. 07.006.

10. Blaylock RL, Strunecka A Immune-glutametric Dysfunction as a central Mechanism of the Autism Spectrum Disorders. Curr Med Chem 2009; 16:157-70.

11. Jyonouchi, H., 2010. Autism spectrum disorders and allergy: observation from a pediatric allergy/immunology clinic. Expert. Rev. Clin. Immunol. 6, 397-411.

12. Chen, M.-H., Su, T.-P., Chen, Y.-S., Hsu, J.-W., Huang, K.-L., Chang, W.-H., et al. (2013). Comorbidity of allergic and autoimmune diseases in patients with autism spectrum disorder: a nationwide population-based study. Res. Autism Spectr. Disord. 7, 205-212. doi: 10.1016/j.rasd.2012.08.008.

13. Kotey, S., Ertel, K., and Whitcomb, B. (2014). Co-occurrence of autism and asthma in a nationally-representative sample of children in the United States. J. Autism Dev. Disord. 44, 3083-3088. doi: 10.1007/s10803-014-2174-y.

14. Shibata, A., Hitomi, Y., Kambayashi, Y., Hibino, Y., Yamazaki, M., Mitoma, J., et al. (2013). Epidemiological study on the involvements of environmental factors and allergy in child mental health using the Autism Screening Questionnaire. Res. Autism Spectr. Disord. 7, 132140. doi: 10.1016/j.rasd.2012.06.003.

15. Mostafa, G. A., Hamza, R. T., and El-Shahawi, H. H. (2008). Allergic manifestations in autistic children: relation to disease severity. J. Pediatr. Neurol. 6, 115-123. doi: 10.1055/s-0035-1557446.

16. Mostafa, G. A., El-Sherif, D. F., and Al-Ayadhi, L. Y. (2014). Systemic auto-antibodies in children with autism. J. Neuroimmunol. 272, 94-98. doi: 10.1016/j.jneuroim.2014.04.011.

17. Mostafa, G. A., and Al-Ayadhi, L. Y. (2015). The possible link between elevated serum levels of epithelial cell-derived neutrophil-activating peptide-78 (ENA-78/CXCL5) and autoimmunity in autistic children. Behav. Brain Funct. 11:11. doi: 10.1186/s12993-015-0056-x.

18. Singh, V.K. Phenotypic expression of autoimmune autistic disorder (AAD): A major subset of autism. Ann. Clin. Psychiatry 2009, 21, 148–161.

19. Mostafa, G. A., and Al-Ayadhi, L. Y. (2012). The relationship between the increased frequency of serum antineuronal antibodies and the severity of autism in children. Eur. J. Paediatr. Neurol. 16, 464-468. doi: 10.1016/j.ejpn.2011.12.010.

20. Mostafa, G. A., and Al-Ayadhi, L. Y. (2013). The possible relationship between allergic manifestations and elevated serum levels of brain specific auto-antibodies in autistic children. J. Neuroimmunol. 261, 77-81. doi: 10.1016/j.jneuroim.2013.04.003.

21. Vojdani, Aristo & Lambert, Jama & Vojdani, Elroy. (2017). Association between environmental triggers and neuroautoimmunity in autism spectrum disorders. 3.

22. Vojdani, A., Campbell, A.W., Anyanwu, E., Kashanian, A., Bock, K., Vojdani, E., 2002. Antibodies to neuron-specific antigens in children with autism: possible cross-reaction with encephalitogenic proteins from milk, Chlamydia pneumoniae and Streptococcus group A. J. Neuroimmunol. 129 (1-2), 168-177.

23. Blaylock, R.L. Excitotoxicity, a possible central mechanism in fluoride neurotoxicity. Fluoride, 2004, 37, 264-77.

24. Strunecka, A.; Patocka, J.; Blaylock, R.L.; Chinoy, N.J. Fluoride interactions: From molecules to disease. Curr. Signal Transd. Ther., 2007, 2, 190-213.

25. Jyonouchi, H., Geng, L., Ruby, A., Zimmerman-Bier, B., 2005. Dysregulated innate immune responses in young children with autism spectrum disorders: their relationship to gastrointestinal symptoms and dietary intervention. Neuropsychobiology 51, 77-85.

26. Genuis, S. J. (2010). Sensitivity-related illness: The escalating pandemic of allergy, food intolerance and chemical sensitivity. Science of The Total Environment, 408(24), 6047-6061. doi:10.1016/j.scitotenv.2010.08.047.

27. Dinan, T. G., Stilling, R. M., Stanton, C., and Cryan, J. F. (2015). Collective unconscious: how gut microbes shape human behavior. J. Psychiatr. Res. 63, 1-9. doi: 10.1016/j.jpsychires.2015.02.021.

28. Coury DL, Ashwood P, Fasano A, et al. Gastrointestinal conditions in children with autism spectrum disorder: developing a research agenda. Pediatrics. 2012;130(Suppl 2):S160-S168.

29. Wu, H. J., and Wu, E. (2012). The role of gut microbiota in immune homeostasis and autoimmunity. Gut Microbes 3, 414. doi: 10.4161/gmic.19320.

30. Williams BL, Hornig M, Buie T, Bauman ML, Cho Paik M, Wick I, et al. Impaired carbohydrate digestion and transport and mucosal dysbiosis in the intestines of children with autism and gastrointestinal disturbances. PLoS ONE (2011) 6:e24585. doi: 10.1371/journal.pone.0024585.

31. Cristiano, C., Lama, A., Lembo, F., Mollica, M. P., Calignano, A., & Mattace Raso, G. (2018). Interplay Between Peripheral and Central Inflammation in Autism Spectrum Disorders: Possible Nutritional and Therapeutic Strategies. Frontiers in Physiology, 9. doi:10.3389/fphys.2018.00184.

32. Vojdani A. Food immune reactivity and neuroautoimmunity. Funct Neurol Rehabil Ergon, 2014; 4(2-3):175-195.

33. Jyonouchi, H., Geng, L., Streck, D. L., & Toruner, G. A. (2011). Children with autism spectrum disorders (ASD) who exhibit chronic gastrointestinal (GI) symptoms and marked fluctuation of behavioral symptoms exhibit distinct innate immune abnormalities and transcriptional profiles of peripheral blood (PB) monocytes. Journal of Neuroimmunology, 238, 73-80.

Chapter Three

1. Adams JB, Johansen LJ, Powell LD, Quig D, Rubin RA. Gastrointestinal flora and gastrointestinal status in children with autism-comparisons to typical children and correlation with autism severity. BMC Gastroenterol 2011;11:22.

2. Finegold SM, Dowd SE, Gontcharova V, Liu C, Henley KE, Wolcott RD, et al. Pyrosequencing study of fecal microflora of autistic and control children. Anaerobe 2010;16:444-53.

3. Song Y, Liu C, Finegold SM. Real-time PCR quantitation of Clostridia in feces of autistic children. Appl Environ Microbiol 2004;70(11):6459-65.

4. Finegold SM. State of the art; microbiology in health and disease. Intestinal bacterial flora in autism. Anaerobe 2011;17:367-8.

5. Finegold SM, Downes J, Summanen PH. Microbiology of regressive autism. Anaerobe 2012;18:260-2.

6. Williams BL, Hornig M, Buie T, et al. Impaired carbohydrate digestion and transport and mucosal dysbiosis in the intestines of children with autism and gastrointestinal disturbances. PLoS One. 2011;6(9):e24585.

7. Wang L, Christophersen CT, Sorich MJ, Gerber JP, Angley MT, Conlon MA. Increased abundance of Sutterella spp. and Ruminococcus torques in feces of children with autism spectrum disorder. Mol Autism. 2013;4(1):42.

8. Wang L, Conlon MA, Christophersen CT, Sorich MJ, Angley MT. Gastrointestinal microbiota and metabolite biomarkers in children with autism spectrum disorders. Biomark Med. 2014;8(3):331-44.

9. Kang DW, Park JG, Ilhan ZE, et al. Reduced incidence of Prevotella and other fermenters in intestinal microflora of autistic children. PLoS One. 2013;8(7):e68322.

10. Krajmalnik-Brown R, Lozupone C, Kang DW, Adams JB. Gut bacteria in children with autism spectrum disorders: challenges and promise of studying how a complex community influences a complex disease. Microb Ecol Health Dis. 2015;26:26914.

11. Bilbo SD, Nevison CD, Parker W. A model for the induction of autism in the ecosystem of the human body: the anatomy of a modern pandemic? Microb Ecol Health Dis. 2015;26:26253.

12. De Angelis M, Piccolo M, Vannini L, et al. Fecal microbiota and metabolome of children with autism and pervasive developmental disorder not otherwise specified. PLoS One. 2013;8(10):e76993.

13. Buie T. Potential etiologic factors of microbiome disruption in autism. Clin Ther. 2015;37(5):976-83.

14. Morris, G., Berk, M., Carvalho, A., Caso, J. R., Sanz, Y., Walder, K., et al. (2017). The role of the microbial metabolites including tryptophan catabolites and short chain fatty acids in the pathophysiology of immune-inflammatory and neuroimmune disease. Mol. Neurobiol. 54, 4432-4451. doi: 10.1007/s12035-016-0004-2.

15. Mezzelani A, Landini M, Facchiano F, Raggi ME, Villa L, Molteni M, et al. Environment, dysbiosis, immunity and sex-specific susceptibility: a translational hypothesis for regressive autism pathogenesis. Nutr Neurosci 2015;18(4):14561. doi:10.1179/1476830513Y.0000000108.

16. MacFabe DF. Short-chain fatty acid fermentation products of the gut microbiome: implications in autism spectrum disorders. Microb Ecol Health Dis 2012; 23: 19260, doi: http://dx.doi.org/10.3402/mehd.v23i0.19260.

17. Wang L, Christophersen CT, Sorich MJ, Gerber JP, Angley MT, Conlon MA. Elevated fecal short chain fatty acid and ammonia concentrations in children with autism spectrum disorder. Dig Dis Sci. (2012) 57:2096102. doi: 10.1007/s10620-012-2167-7.

18. Frye RE, Melnyk S, Macfabe DF. Unique acyl-carnitine profiles are potential biomarkers for acquired mitochondrial disease in autism spectrum disorder. Transl Psychiatry 2013; 3: e220.

19. Frye, Richard & Rose, Shannon & Slattery, John & MacFabe, Derrick. (2015). Gastrointestinal dysfunction in autism spectrum disorder: the role of the mitochondria and the enteric microbiome. Microbial ecology in health and disease. 26. 27458. 10.3402/mehd.v26.27458.

20. MacFabe DF, Cain DP, Rodriguez-Capote K, Franklin AE, Hoffman JE, Boon F, et al. Neurobiological effects of intraventricular propionic acid in rats: possible role of short chain fatty acids on the pathogenesis and characteristics of autism spectrum disorders. Behav Brain Res 2007; 176: 149-69.

21. Brock M, Buckel W. On the mechanism of action of the antifungal agent propionate. Eur J Biochem 2004; 271: 3227-41.

22. Jyonouchi, H., Geng, L., Ruby, A., Zimmerman-Bier, B., 2005. Dysregulated innate immune responses in young children with autism spectrum disorders: their relationship to gastrointestinal symptoms and dietary intervention. Neuropsychobiology 51, 77-85.

23. Vojdani A. Food immune reactivity and neuroautoimmunity. Funct Neurol Rehabil Ergon, 2014; 4(2-3):175-195.

24. Vojdani, Aristo & Lambert, Jama & Vojdani, Elroy. (2017). Blood-based markers in autism spectrum disorders Blood-based markers in autism spectrum disorders. Internal Medicine. 3.

25. Buie, T. (2015). Potential Etiologic Factors of Microbiome Disruption in Autism. Clinical Therapeutics, 37(5), 976–983. doi:10.1016/j.clinthera.2015.04.001.

26. Atarashi K, Tanoue T, Shima T, et al. Induction of colonic regulatory T cells by indigenous Clostridium species. Science. 2011;331:337-341.

27. Finegold SM, Molitoris D, Song Y et al. Gastrointestinal microflora studies in late-onset autism. Clin Infect Dis 2002; 35 (Suppl 1): S6-S16.

28. Parracho HM, Bingham MO, Gibson GR, McCartney AL. Differences between the gut microflora of children with autistic spectrum disorders and that of healthy children. J Med Microbiol. (2005) 54(Pt 10):98791. doi: 10.1099/jmm.0.46101-0.

29. Shaw W. Increased urinary excretion of a 3-(3-hydroxyphenyl)-3-hydroxypropionic acid (HPHPA), an abnormal phenylalanine metabolite of Clostridia spp. in the gastrointestinal tract, in urine samples from patients with autism and schizophrenia. Nutr Neurosci 2010;13:135-43.

30. Finegold SM. Therapy and epidemiology of autism-clostridial spores as key elements. Med Hypotheses 2008;70:508-11.

31. Bolte E. Autism and Clostridium tetani. Med Hypotheses 1998; 51:133-144.

32. Persico, A.M., & Napolioni, V. (2013). Urinary p-cresol in autism spectrum disorder. Neurotoxicology and Teratology, 36, 82-90.

33. Selmer, T., & Andrei, P. I. (2001). p-Hydroxyphenylacetate decarboxylase from Clostridium difficile. European Journal of Biochemistry, 268(5), 1363–1372. doi:10.1046/j.1432-1327.2001.02001.x.

34. Goodhart, P. J., DeWolf, W. E., & Kruse, L. I. (1987). Mechanism-based inactivation of dopamine .beta.-hydroxylase by p-cresol and related alkylphenols. Biochemistry, 26(9), 2576–2583. doi:10.1021/bi00383a025.

35. Gabriele S, Sacco R, Altieri L, Neri C, Urbani A, Bravaccio C, Riccio MP, Iovene MR, Bombace F, deMagistris L, Persico AM. Slow intestinal transit contributes to elevate urinary p-cresol level in Italian autistic children. Autism Res. 2015;. doi:10.1002/aur.1571.

36. Altieri L, Neri C, Sacco R, Curatolo P, Benvenuto A, Muratori F, et al. Urinary p-cresol is elevated in small children with severe autism spectrum disorder. Biomarkers (2011) 16:25260. doi:10.3109/1354750X.2010.548010.

37. Gabriele S, Sacco R, Cerullo S, Neri C, Urbani A, Tripi G, et al. Urinary p-cresol is elevated in young French children with autism spectrum disorder: a replication study. Biomarkers(2014) 19:46370. doi: 10.3109/1354750X.2014.936911.

38. Keşli, R., Gökçen, C., Buluğ, U., & Terzi, Y. (2014). Investigation of the relation between anaerobic bacteria genus clostridium and late-onset autism etiology in children. Journal of immunoassay & immunochemistry. 35. 101-9. 10.1080/15321819.2013.792834.

39. Frye RE, Melnyk S, Macfabe DF. Unique acyl-carnitine profiles are potential biomarkers for acquired mitochondrial disease in autism spectrum disorder. Transl Psychiatry 2013; 3: e220.

40. François L. Mayer, et. Al. Candida albicans pathogenicity mechanisms. Virulence . Feb 15, 2013; 4(2): 119-128.

41. Strati F, Cavalieri D, Albanese D, De Felice C, Donati C, Hayek J, et al. New evidences on the altered gut microbiota in autism spectrum disorders. Microbiome (2017) 5:24. doi: 10.1186/s40168-017-0242-1.

42. Kantarcioglu AS, Kiraz N, Aydin A. Microbiota-gut-brain axis: yeast species isolated from stool samples of children with suspected or diagnosed autism spectrum disorders and in vitro susceptibility against nystatin and fluconazole. Mycopathologia (2016) 181:17. doi: 10.1007/s11046-015-9949-3.

43. Iovene MR, Bombace F, Maresca R, Sapone A, Iardino P, Picardi A, et al. Intestinal dysbiosis and yeast isolation in stool of subjects with autism spectrum disorders. Mycopathologia (2017) 182:34963. Doi: 10.1007/s11046-016-0068-6.

44. Noto A, Fanos V, Barberini L, Grapov D, Fattuoni C, Zaffanello M, et al. The urinary metabolomics profile of an Italian autistic children population and their unaffected siblings. J Matern Fetal Neonatal Med. (2014) 27(sup2):46-52. doi: 10.3109/14767058.2014.954784.

45. Kaluzna-Czaplinska J, Blaszczyk S. The level of arabinitol in autistic children after probiotic therapy. Nutrition (2012) 28:1246.doi: 10.1016/j.nut.2011.08.002.

46. Hughes HK, Ashwood P. Anti-Candida albicans IgG Antibodies in Children With Autism Spectrum Disorders. Frontiers in Psychiatry. 2018; 9:627. https://doi.org/10.3389/fpsyt.2018.00627.

47. De Santis, B., Raggi, M., Moretti, G., Facchiano, F., Mezzelani, A., Villa, L., ... Brera, C. (2017). Study on the Association among Mycotoxins and

other Variables in Children with Autism. Toxins, 9(7), 203. doi:10.3390/toxins9070203.

48. De Santis, B., Brera, C., Mezzelani, A., Soricelli, S., Ciceri, F., Moretti, G., ... Raggi, M. E. (2017). Role of mycotoxins in the pathobiology of autism: A first evidence. Nutritional Neuroscience, 1–13. doi:10.1080/1028415x.2017.1357793.

49. Duringer J, Fombonne E, Craig M. No association between mycotoxin exposure and autism: a pilot case-control study in school-aged children. Toxins 2016;8(7):224.

50. Williams JH, Phillips TD, Jolly PE, Stiles JK, Jolly CM, Aggarwal D. Human aflatoxicosis in developing countries: a review of toxicology, exposure, potential health consequences, and interventions. Am J Clin Nutr 2004;80:1106-22.

51. Wild CP, Gong YY. Mycotoxins and human disease: a largely ignored global health issue. Carcinogenesis 2010;31(1):71-82. doi:10.1093/carcin/bgp264.

52. Liu BH, Wu TS, Yu FY, Su CC. Induction of oxidative stress response by the mycotoxin patulin in mammalian cells. Toxicol Sci. 2007;95(2):340-7. doi: 10.1093/toxsci/kfl156.

53. Doi K, Uetsuka K. Mechanisms of mycotoxin-induced neurotoxicity through oxidative stress-associated pathways. Int J Mol Sci. 2011;12(8):5213-37. doi: 10.3390/ijms12085213.

54. Puel O, Galtier P, Oswald IP. Biosynthesis and toxicological effects of patulin. Toxins 2010;2:613-31.

Chapter Four

1. Schreck KA, Williams K, Smith AF (2004) A comparison of eating behaviors between children with and without autism. J Autism Dev Disord 34:433–438.

2. Bandini LG, Anderson SE, Curtin C, et al. Food selectivity in children with autism spectrum disorders and typically developing children. J Pediatr. 2010;157(2):259-264.

3. Zimmer, Michelle & Hart, Laura & Manning-Courtney, Patricia & Murray, Donna & Bing, Nicole & Summer, Suzanne. (2011). Food Variety as a Predictor of Nutritional Status Among Children with Autism. Journal of autism and developmental disorders. 42. 549-56. 10.1007/s10803-011-1268-z.

4. Adams, J.B.; Audhya, T.; McDonough-Means, S.; Rubin, R.A.; Quig, D.; Geis, E.; Gehn, E.; Loresto, M.; Mitchell, J.; Atwood, S.; et al. Nutritional and Metabolic Status of Children with Autism vs. Neurotypical Children, and the Association with Autism Severity. Nutr. Metab. 2011, 8, 34.

5. Goyer RA Toxic and Essential Metal Interactions. Ann Rev of Nutr 1997; 17: 37-50.

6. Goyer, R. A. (1995). Nutrition and metal toxicity. The American Journal of Clinical Nutrition, 61(3), 646S–650S. doi:10.1093/ajcn/61.3.646s.

7. Hyman SL, Steward PA, Schmidt B, et al. (2012) Nutrient intake from food which autism. Pediatrics 103(Suppl. 2): 145-153.

8. Coury, Daniel & Ashwood, Paul & Fasano, Alessio & Fuchs, George & Geraghty, Maureen & Kaul, Ajay & Mawe, Gary & Patterson, Paul & Jones, Nancy. (2012). Gastrointestinal Conditions in Children With Autism Spectrum Disorder: Developing a Research Agenda. PEDIATRICS. 130. S160-S168. 10.1542/peds.2012-0900N.

9. Xia W et al., A preliminary study on nutritional status and intake in Chinese children with autism. Eur J Pediatr 2010, 69(10):1201-6.

10. Altenburger J, Geraghty ME, Wolf K, Taylor CA, Lane AE. The quality of nutritional intake in children with autism. J Am Diet Assoc. 2010;110(9):A40.

11. Meguid, N.A.; Anwar, M.; Bjørklund, G.; Hashish, A.; Chirumbolo, S.; Hemimi, M.; Sultan, E. Dietary adequacy of Egyptian children with autism spectrum disorder compared to healthy developing children. Metab. Brain Dis. 2017, 32, 607–615.

12. Marí-Bauset, Salvador & Llopis-González, Agustín & Zazpe, Itziar & Mari-Sanchis, Amelia & Morales-Suárez-Varela, Maria. (2016). Comparison of nutritional status between children with autism spectrum disorder and typically developing children in the Mediterranean Region (Valencia, Spain). Autism. 21. 10.1177/1362361316636976.

13. Osredkar J, Sustar N (2011) Copper and Zinc, Biological Role and Significance of Copper/Zinc Imbalance. J Clinic Toxicol S3:001. doi:10.4172/2161-0494.S3-001.

14. Faber S, Zinn GM, Kern JC 2nd, et al. The Plasma Zinc/Serum Copper ratio as a biomarker in Children with Autism Spectrum Disorders. Biomarkers 2009; 14:171-180.

15. Priya MD, Geetha A Level of Trace Elements (Copper, Zinc, Magnesium and Selenium) and Toxic Elements (Lead and Mercury) in the Hair and Nail of Children with Autism. Biol Trace Ele Res 2010:1-11.

16. Madsen E, Gitlin JD Copper and Iron Disorders of the Brain. Annu Rev Neurosci 2007; 30:17-337.

17. Li, Si-Ou & Wang, Jia-Liang & Bjorklund, Geir & Zhao, Wei-Na & Yin, Chang-Hao. (2014). Serum copper and zinc levels in individuals with autism spectrum disorders. Neuroreport. 25. 10.1097/WNR.0000000000000251.

18. Russo AJ, Bazin AP, Bigega R, Carlson RS 3rd, Cole MG, Contreras DC, et al. Plasma copper and zinc concentration in individuals with autism correlate with selected symptom severity. Nutr Metab Insights 2012; 5:41-47.

19. Elsheshtawy, E., Tobar, S., Sherra, K., Atallah, S., Elkasaby, R., 2011. Study of some biomarkers in hair of children with autism. Middle East Curr. Psychiatry 18 (1), 6-10.

20. Meguid, N. A., Bjørklund, G., Gebril, O. H., Doşa, M. D., Anwar, M., Elsaeid, A., ... Chirumbolo, S. (2019). The role of zinc supplementation on the metallothionein system in children with autism spectrum disorder. Acta Neurologica Belgica. doi:10.1007/s13760-019-01181-9.

21. Russo AJ, deVito R (2011) Analysis of copper and zinc plasma concentration the efficacy of zinc therapy in individuals with Asperger's syndrome, pervasive developmental disorder not otherwise specified (PDD-NOS) and autism. Biomark Insights 6:127–133.

22. Russo AJ. Increased Copper in Individuals with Autism Normalizes Post Zinc Therapy More Efficiently in Individuals with Concurrent GI Disease. Nutrition and Metabolic Insights 2011;4: 49-54.

23. Mazahery, Hajar & Camargo, Carlos & Conlon, Cath & Beck, Kathryn & Kruger, Marlena & Von Hurst, Pamela. (2016). Vitamin D and Autism Spectrum Disorder: A Literature Review. Nutrients. 8. 236. 10.3390/nu8040236.

24. Fernell, E.; Bejerot, S.; Westerlund, J.; Miniscalco, C.; Simila, H.; Eyles, D.; Gillberg, C.; Humble, M.B. Autism Spectrum Disorder and low vitamin D at birth: A sibling control study. Mol. Autism 2015, 6, 3.

25. Kocovska, E.; Andorsdottir, G.; Weihe, P.; Halling, J.; Fernell, E.; Stora, T.; Biskupsto, R.; Gillberg, I.C.; Shea, R.; Billstedt, E.; et al. Vitamin D in the general population of young adults with autism in the faroe islands. J. Autism Dev. Disord. 2014, 44, 2996-3005.

26. Gong, Z.L.; Luo, C.M.; Wang, L.; Shen, L.; Wei, F.; Tong, R.J.; Liu, Y. Serum 25-hydroxyvitamin D levels in Chinese children with Autism Spectrum Disorders. Neuroreport 2014, 25, 2327.

27. Feng, J.; Shan, L.; Du, L.; Wang, B.; Li, H.; Wang, W.; Wang, T.; Dong, H.; Yue, X.; Xu, Z.; et al. Clinical improvement following vitamin D3 supplementation in Autism Spectrum Disorder. Nutr. Neurosci. 2016.

28. Meguid, N.A.; Hashish, A.F.; Anwar, M.; Sidhom, G. Reduced serum levels of 25-hydroxy and 1,25-dihydroxy vitamin D in egyptian children with autism. J. Altern. Complement. Med. (New York NY) 2010, 16, 641-645.

29. Mostafa, G.A.; Al-Ayadhi, L.Y. Reduced serum concentrations of 25-hydroxy vitamin D in children with autism: Relation to autoimmunity. J. Neuroinflamm. 2012, 9, 201.

30. Bener, A.; Khattab, A.O.; Al-Dabbagh, M.M. Is high prevalence of vitamin D deficiency evidence for autism disorder? In a highly endogamous population. J. Pediatr. Neurosci. 2014, 9, 227-233.

31. Saad, K.; Abdel-Rahman, A.A.; Elserogy, Y.M.; Al-Atram, A.A.; Cannell, J.J.; Bjorklund, G.; Abdel-Reheim, M.K.; Othman, H.A.; El-Houfey, A.A.; Abd El-Aziz, N.H.; et al. Vitamin D status in Autism Spectrum Disorders and the efficacy of vitamin D supplementation in autistic children. Nutr. Neurosci. 2015.

32. Desoky, T., Hassan, M. H., Fayed, H. M., and Sakhr, H. M. (2017). Biochemical assessments of thyroid profile, serum 25-hydroxycholecalciferol and cluster of differentiation 5 expression levels among children with autism. Neuropsychiatr. Dis. Treat. 13, 2397-2403. doi: 10.2147/NDT.S146152.

33. Neumeyer, A.M.; Gates, A.; Ferrone, C.; Lee, H.; Misra, M. Bone density in peripubertal boys with Autism Spectrum Disorders. J. Autism Dev. Disord. 2013, 43, 1623-1629.

34. Alvarez, J.A.; Chowdhury, R.; Jones, D.P.; Martin, G.S.; Brigham, K.L.; Binongo, J.N.; Ziegler, T.R.; Tangpricha, V. Vitamin D status is independently associated with plasma glutathione and cysteine thiol/disulphide redox status in adults. Clin. Endocrinol. 2014, 81, 458–466.

35. Codoner-Franch, P.; Tavarez-Alonso, S.; Simo-Jorda, R.; Laporta-Martin, P.; Carratala-Calvo, A.; Alonso-Iglesias, E. Vitamin D status is linked to biomarkers of oxidative stress, inflammation, and endothelial activation in obese children. J. Pediatr. 2012, 161, 848–854.

36. Mazahery, H.; Stonehouse, W.; Delshad, M.; Kruger, M.C.; Conlon, C.A.; Beck, K.L.; von Hurst, P.R. Relationship between Long Chain n-3 Polyunsaturated Fatty Acids and Autism Spectrum Disorder: Systematic Review and Meta-Analysis of Case-Control and Randomised Controlled Trials. Nutrients 2017, 9, 155.

37. S. Vancassel et al., Plasma fatty acid levels in autistic children, Prostaglandins Leukot Essent Fatty Acids 2001 65:1-7.

38. Bell et al Essential fatty acids and phospholipase A2 in autistic spectrum disorders. Prostaglandins Leukot Essent Fatty Acids. 2004 Oct;71(4):201-4.

39. Wiest et al Plasma fatty acid profiles in autism: a case-control study Prostaglandins Leukot Essent Fatty Acids. 2009 Apr;80(4):221-7.

40. Bell et al 2010, The fatty acid compositions of erythrocyte and plasma polar lipids in children with autism, developmental delay or typically developing controls and the effect of fish oil intake. Br. J. Nutri. 103 1160-7.

41. Latif A, Heinz P, Cook R: Iron Deficiency in Autism and Asperger Syndrome. Autism 2002, 6:103.

42. Dosman CF, Drmic IE, Brian JA, Senthilselvan A, Harford M, Smith R, Roberts SW: Ferritin as an indicator of suspected iron deficiency in children with autism spectrum disorder: prevalence of low serum ferritin concentration. Dev Med Child Neurol 2006, 48(12):1008-9.

43. Järup, L., Åkesson, A., 2009. Current status of cadmium as an environmental health problem. Toxicol. Appl. Pharmacol. 238 (3), 201-208.

44. Grigg-Damberger M, Ralls F. Treatment strategies for complex behavioral insomnia in children with neurodevelopmental disorders. Curr Opin Pulm Med, 2013;19:616-625.

45. Frye, Richard & Rose, Shannon & Slattery, John & MacFabe, Derrick. (2015). Gastrointestinal dysfunction in autism spectrum disorder: the role of the mitochondria and the enteric microbiome. Microbial ecology in health and disease. 26. 27458. 10.3402/mehd.v26.27458.

46. Frye RE, Rossignol DA. Mitochondrial dysfunction can connect the diverse medical symptoms associated with autism spectrum disorders. Pediatr Res 2011; 69: 41R-7R.

47. Rossignol DA, Frye RE. Mitochondrial dysfunction in autism spectrum disorders: a systematic review and meta-analysis. Mol Psychiatry 2012; 17: 290-314.

48. Frye RE. Biomarkers of abnormal energy metabolism in children with autism spectrum disorder. N Am J Med Sci 2012; 5: 141-7.

49. Weissman, J.R.; Kelley, R.I.; Bauman,M.L.; Cohen, B.H.;Murray, K.F.;Mitchell, R.L.; Kern, R.L.; Natowicz,M.R. Mitochondrial disease in

autism spectrum disorder patients: A cohort analysis. PLoS ONE 2008, 3, e3815.

50. Oliveira, G.; Ataíde, A.; Marques, C.; Miguel, T.S.; Coutinho, A.M.; Mota-Vieira, L.; Goncalves, E.; Lopes, N.M.; Rodrigues, V.; Carmona da Mota, H.; et al. Epidemiology of autism spectrum disorder in Portugal: Prevalence, clinical characterization, and medical conditions. Dev. Med. Child Neurol. 2007, 49, 726–733.

51. Oliveira, G.; Diogo, L.; Grazina, M.; Garcia, P.; Ataíde, A.; Marques, C.; Miguel, T.; Borges, L.; Vicente, A.M.; Oliveira, C.R. Mitochondrial dysfunction in autism spectrum disorders: A population-based study. Dev. Med. Child Neurol. 2005, 47, 185–189.

52. Correia, C.; Coutinho, A.M.; Diogo, L.; Grazina, M.; Marques, C.; Miguel, T.; Ataíde, A.; Almeida, J.; Borges, L.; Oliveira, C.; et al. Brief report: High frequency of biochemical markers for mitochondrial dysfunction in autism: No association with the mitochondrial aspartate/glutamate carrier SLC25A12 gene. J. Autism Dev. Disord. 2006, 36, 1137–1140.

53. Mostafa GA, El-Gamal HA, El-Wakkad ASE, El-Shorbagy OE, Hamza MM. Polyunsaturated fatty acids, carnitine and lactate as biological markers of brain energy in autistic children. Int J Child Neuropsychiatry 2005; 2: 179-188.

54. Filipek PA, Juranek J, Smith M, Mays LZ, Ramos ER, Bocian M, et al. Mitochondrial dysfunction in autistic patients with 15q inverted duplication. Ann Neurol 2003; 53: 801-4.

55. Filipek, P.A.; Juranek, J.; Nguyen, M.T.; Cummings, C.; Gargus, J.J. Relative carnitine deficiency in autism. J. Autism Dev. Disord 2004, 34, 615–623.

56. Geier DA, Kern JK, Garver CR, Adams JB, Audhya T, Geier MR: A prospective study of transsulfuration biomarkers in autistic disorders. Neurochem Res 2009, 34(2):386-93, Erratum in: Neurochem Res. 2009, 34(2):394.

57. Geier, D. A., Kern, J. K., Garver, C. R., Adams, J. B., Audhya, T., Nataf, R., & Geier, M. R. (2009). Biomarkers of environmental toxicity and susceptibility in autism. Journal of the Neurological Sciences, 280(1-2), 101–108. doi:10.1016/j.jns.2008.08.021

58. James SJ, Cutler P, Melnyk S, Jernigan S, Janak L, Gaylor DW, Neubrander JA: Metabolic biomarkers of increased oxidative stress and impaired methylation capacity in children with autism. Am J Clin Nutr 2004, 80(6):1611-7.

59. James SJ, Melnyk S, Jernigan S, Cleves MA, Halsted CH, Wong DH, Cutler P, Bock K, Boris M, Bradstreet JJ, Baker SM, Gaylor DW: Metabolic endophenotype and related genotypes are associated with oxidative stress in children with autism. Am J Med Genet B Neuropsychiatr Genet 2006, 141:947-956.

60. James SJ, Melnyk S, Fuchs G, Reid T, Jernigan S, Pavliv O, Hubanks A, Gaylor DW: Efficacy of methylcobalamin and folinic acid treatment on glutathione redox status in children with autism. Am J Clin Nutr 2009, 89(1):425-30.

61. Rossignol, D.A.; Frye, R.E. Evidence linking oxidative stress, mitochondrial dysfunction, and inflammation in the brain of individuals with autism. Front. Physiol. 2014, 5, 150.

62. Ghezzo, A.; Visconti, P.; Abruzzo, P.M.; Bolotta, A.; Ferreri, C.; Gobbi, G.; Malisardi, G.; Manfredini, S.; Marini, M.; Nanetti, L.; et al. Oxidative stress and erythrocyte membrane alterations in children with autism: Correlation with clinical features. PLoS ONE 2013, 8, e66418.

63. Melnyk S, Fuchs GJ, Schulz E, et al. Metabolic imbalance associated with methylation dysregulation and oxidative damage in children with autism. J Autism Dev Disord. 2012;42(3):367–77.

64. Rose, S.; Melnyk, S.; Pavliv, O.; Bai, S.; Nick, T.G.; Frye, R.E.; James, S.J. Evidence of oxidative damage and inflammation associated with low glutathione redox status in the autism brain. Transl. Psychiatry 2012, 2, e134.

65. Al-Gadani, Y., El-Ansary, A., Attas, O., Al-Ayadhi, L., 2009. Metabolic biomarkersrelated to oxidative stress and antioxidant status in Saudi autistic children.Clin. Biochem. 42, 1032–1040.

66. Al-Yafee, Y.A., Al-Ayadhi, L.Y., Haq, S.H., El-Ansary, A.K., 2011. Novel metabolic biomarkers related to sulfur-dependent detoxification pathways in autistic patients of Saudi Arabia. BMC Neurol. 11, 139.

67. Han, Y., Xi, Q.Q., Dai, W., Yang, S.H., Gao, L., Su, Y.Y., et al., 2015. Abnormal transsulfuration metabolism and reduced antioxidant capacity in Chinese children with autism spectrum disorders. Int. J. Dev. Neurosci. 46, 27–32.

68. Paşca, S.P., Dronca, E., Kaucsár, T., Craciun, E.C., Endreffy, E., Ferencz, B.K., et al.,2009. One carbon metabolism disturbances and the C677T MTHFR gene polymprhism in children with autism spectrum disorders. J. Cell Mol. Med. 13,4229–4238.

69. Frye RE, Melnyk S, Macfabe DF. Unique acyl-carnitine profiles are potential biomarkers for acquired mitochondrial disease in autism spectrum disorder. Transl Psychiatry 2013; 3: e220.

70. Adams, James & Audhya, Tapan & McDonough-Means, Sharon & Rubin, Robert & Quig, David & Geis, Elizabeth & Gehn, Eva & Loresto, Melissa & Mitchell, Jessica & Atwood, Sharon & Barnhouse, Suzanne & Lee, Wondra. (2011). Effect of a vitamin/mineral supplement on children and adults with autism. BMC pediatrics. 11. 111. 10.1186/1471-2431-11-111.

71. Blaylock RL, Strunecka A Immune-glutametric Dysfunction as A central Mechanism of the Autism Spectrum Disorders. Curr Med Chem 2009; 16:157-70.

72. Zheng, Z., Zhu, T., Qu, Y., & Mu, D. (2016). Blood Glutamate Levels in Autism Spectrum Disorder: A Systematic Review and Meta-Analysis. PLOS ONE, 11(7), e0158688. doi:10.1371/journal.pone.0158688.

73. Rojas, D. C. (2014). The role of glutamate and its receptors in autism and the use of glutamate receptor antagonists in treatment. Journal of Neural Transmission, 121(8), 891–905. doi:10.1007/s00702-014-1216-0.

74. Shimmura, Chie & Suda, Shiro & Tsuchiya, Kenji & Hashimoto, Kenji & Ohno, Koji & Matsuzaki, Hideo & Iwata, Keiko & Matsumoto, Kaori &

Wakuda, Tomoyasu & Kameno, Yosuke & Suzuki, Katsuaki & Tsujii, Masatsugu & Nakamura, Kazuhiko & Takei, Nori & Mori, Norio. (2011). Alteration of Plasma Glutamate and Glutamine Levels in Children with High-Functioning Autism. PloS one. 6. e25340. 10.1371/journal.pone.0025340.

75. Blaylock, R.L. Excitotoxicity, a possible central mechanism in fluoride neurotoxicity. Fluoride, 2004, 37, 264-77.

76. Geier DA, King PG, Sykes LK, Geier MR. A comprehensive review of mercury provoked autism. Indian J Med Res 2008; 128:383-411.

77. Adams, James & Audhya, Tapan & Geis, Elizabeth & Gehn, Eva & Fimbres, Valeria & Pollard, Elena & Mitchell, Jessica & Ingram, Julie & Hellmers, Robert & Laake, Dana & Matthews, Julie & Li, Kefeng & Naviaux, Jane & Naviaux, Robert & Adams, Rebecca & Coleman, Devon & Quig, David. (2018). Comprehensive Nutritional and Dietary Intervention for Autism Spectrum Disorder--A Randomized, Controlled 12-Month Trial. Nutrients. 10. 369. 10.3390/nu10030369.

78. Waring RH, Ngong JM, Klovsra L, Green S, Sharp H: Biochemical Parameters in Autistic Children. Dev Brain Dysfunct 1997, 10:40-43.

79. O'Reilly, B.A.; Warning, R.H. Enzyme and Sulphur Oxidation Deficiencies in Autistic Children with Known Food/Chemical Sensitivities. J. Orthomol. Med. 1993, 8, 198–200.

80. Alberti, A.; Pirrone, P.; Elia, M.;Waring, R.H.; Romano, C. Sulphation deficit in "low-functioning" autistic children: A pilot study. Biol. Psychiatry 1999, 46, 420–424.

81. Horvath, K.; Perman, J.A. Autistic disorder and gastrointestinal disease. Curr. Opin. Pediatr. 2002, 14, 583–587.

82. Waring, R.H.; Klovrsa, L.V. Sulfur Metabolism in Autism. J. Nutr. Environ. Med. 2000, 10, 25–32.

83. Konstantynowicz J, Porowski T, Zoch-Zwierz W, et al. A potential pathogenic role of oxalate in autism. Eur J Paediatr Neurol. 2012;16(5):485-491.

Chapter Five

1. Genuis, S. J., & Kyrillos, E. (2017). The chemical disruption of human metabolism. Toxicology Mechanisms and Methods, 27(7), 477–500. doi:10.1080/15376516.2017.1323986.

2. Grandjean, P., Landrigan, P.J., 2006. Developmental neurotoxicity of industrial chemicals. Lancet 368, 2167–2178.

3. Boggess, Andrew & Faber, Scott & Kern II, John & Kingston, H. M. Skip. (2016). Mean serum-level of common organic pollutants is predictive of behavioral severity in children with autism spectrum disorders. Scientific reports. 6. 26185. 10.1038/srep26185.

4. Priya MD, Geetha A Level of Trace Elements (Copper, Zinc, Magnesium and Selenium) and Toxic Elements (Lead and Mercury) in the Hair and Nail of Children with Autism. Biol Trace Ele Res 2010:1-11.

5. Saghazadeh, Amene & Rezaei, Nima. (2017). Systematic review and meta-analysis links autism and toxic metals and highlights the impact of country development status: Higher blood and erythrocyte levels for mercury and lead, and higher hair antimony, cadmium, lead, and mercury. Progress in Neuro-Psychopharmacology and Biological Psychiatry. 79. 10.1016/j.pnpbp.2017.07.011.

6. Blaurock-Busch, E., Amin, O.R., Dessoki, H.H., Rabah, T., 2012. Toxic metals and essential elements in hair and severity of symptoms among children with autism. Maedica 7 (1), 38-48.

7. Adams, J.B., Audhya, T., McDonough-Means, S., Rubin, R.A., Quig, D., Geis, E., et al., 2013. Toxicological status of children with autism vs. neuro-typical children and the association with autism severity. Biol. Trace Elem. Res. 151 (2), 171-180.

8. Rossignol DA, Genuis SJ, Frye RE. Environmental toxicants and autism spectrum disorders: a systematic review. Transl Psychiatry, Feb 2014; 4:e360.

9. Adams, J.B., Baral, M., Geis, E., Mitchell, J., Ingram, J., Hensley, A., et al., 2009. The severity of autism is associated with toxic metal body burden and red blood cell glutathione levels. J. Toxicol. 2009, 532640.

10. Elsheshtawy, E., Tobar, S., Sherra, K., Atallah, S., Elkasaby, R., 2011. Study of some biomarkers in hair of children with autism. Middle East Curr. Psychiatry 18 (1), 6-10.

11. D. A. Geier, J. K. Kern, C. R. Garver, et al., "Biomarkers of environmental toxicity and susceptibility in autism," Journal of the Neurological Sciences, vol. 280, no. 1-2, pp. 101-108, 2009.

12. Agency for Toxic Substances and Disease Registry, 2019. The priority list of hazardous substances, 2019. Atlanta, GA: U.S. Department of Health and Human Services, Public Health Services 2019 [(http://www.atsdr.cdc.gov/spl/). Accessed 27 October 2019].

13. Risher JF, De Rosa CT. Inorganic: the other mercury. J Environ Health 2007; 70(4):9-16.

14. Tchounwou, P.B., Ayensu, W.K., Ninashvili, N., Sutton, D., 2003. Review: environmental exposure to mercury and its toxicopathologic implications for public health. Environ. Toxicol. 18 (3), 149-175.

15. Geier DA, King PG, Sykes LK, Geier MR. A comprehensive review of mercury provoked autism. Indian J Med Res 2008; 128:383-411.

16. Vojdani, Aristo & Lambert, Jama & Vojdani, Elroy. (2017). Blood-based markers in autism spectrum disorders Blood-based markers in autism spectrum disorders. Internal Medicine. 3.

17. Blaylock RL, Strunecka A Immune-glutametric Dysfunction as A central Mechanism of the Autism Spectrum Disorders. Curr Med Chem 2009; 16:157-70

18. Rice KM, Walker, Jr EM, Wu M, et al. Environmental mercury and its toxic effects. J Prev Med Public Health, 2014; 47(2):74-83.

19. Vojdani, Aristo & Lambert, Jama & Vojdani, Elroy. (2017). Association between environmental triggers and neuroautoimmunity in autism spectrum disorders. 3.

20. Blaylock, R.L. Excitotoxicity, a possible central mechanism in fluoride neurotoxicity. Fluoride, 2004, 37, 264-77.

21. Rodríguez-Barranco, M., Lacasaña, M., Aguilar-Garduño, C., Alguacil, J., Gil, F., González-Alzaga, B., et al., 2013. Association of arsenic, cadmium and manganese exposure with neurodevelopment and behavioural disorders in children: a systematic review and meta-analysis. Sci. Total Environ. 454-455, 562-577.

22. Vahidnia, A., Van der Voet, G.B., De Wolff, F.A., 2007. Arsenic neurotoxicity-a review. Hum. Exp. Toxicol. 26 (10), 823-832.

23. Brockel BJ, Cory-Slechta DA Lead, Attention and Impulsive behavior. Pharmacol Biochem Behav 1998; 60:545-552.

24. Goyer RA Toxic and Essential Metal Interactions. Ann Rev of Nutr 1997; 17: 37-50.

25. Goyer, R. A. (1995). Nutrition and metal toxicity. The American Journal of Clinical Nutrition, 61(3), 646S-650S. doi:10.1093/ajcn/61.3.646s.

26. Méndez-Armenta, M., Ríos, C., 2007. Cadmium neurotoxicity. Environ. Toxicol. Pharmacol. 23 (3), 350-358.

27. Järup, L., Åkesson, A., 2009. Current status of cadmium as an environmental health problem. Toxicol. Appl. Pharmacol. 238 (3), 201-208.

28. https://archive.senseaboutscience.org/data/files/VoYS/Glyphosate_in_our_bread.pdf

29. https://sustainablepulse.com/2016/02/25/german-beer-industry-in-shock-over-probable-carcinogen-glyphosate-contamination

30. Beecham JE, Seneff S (2015) The Possible Link between Autism and Glyphosate Acting as Glycine Mimetic - A Review of Evidence from the Literature with Analysis. J Mol Genet Med 9: 187. doi:10.4172/1747-0862.1000187.

31. Samsel, Anthony & Seneff, Stephanie. (2015). Glyphosate, pathways to modern diseases III: manganese, neurological diseases, and associated pathologies. 6.

32. Samsel, Anthony & Seneff, Stephanie. (2015). Glyphosate, pathways to modern diseases IV: cancer and related pathologies. Journal of Biological Physics and Chemistry. 15. 121-159. 10.4024/11SA15R.jbpc.15.03.

33. Samsel, Anthony & Seneff, Stephanie. (2017). Glyphosate pathways to modern diseases VI: Prions, amyloidoses and autoimmune neurological diseases. Journal of Biological Physics and Chemistry. 17. 8-32. 10.4024/25SA16A.jbpc.17.01.

34. https://www.iarc.fr/wp-content/uploads/2018/07/MonographVolume112-1.pdf

35. https://sustainablepulse.com/2019/05/28/glyphosate-herbicides-now-banned-or-restricted-in-17-countries-worldwide-sustainable-pulse-research/

36. https://www.epa.gov/newsreleases/epa-takes-next-step-review-process-herbicide-glyphosate-reaffirms-no-risk-public-health

37. Rauh, Virginia & Garfinkel, Robin & Perera, Frederica & Andrews, Howard & Hoepner, Lori & Barr, Dana & Whitehead Jr, Ralph & Tang, Deliang & Whyatt, Robin. (2006). Impact of Prenatal Chlorpyrifos Exposure

on Neurodevelopment in the First 3 Years of Life Among Inner-City Children. Pediatrics. 118. e1845-59. 10.1542/peds.2006-0338.

38. https://www.epa.gov/sites/production/files/2017-03/documents/chlorpyrifos3b_order_denying_panna_and_nrdc27s_petitition_to_revoke_tolerances.pdf

39. https://www.nytimes.com/2017/03/29/us/politics/epa-insecticide-chlorpyrifos.html

40. Shelton, Janie & Hertz-Picciotto, Irva & Pessah, Isaac. (2012). Tipping the Balance of Autism Risk: Potential Mechanisms Linking Pesticides and Autism. Environmental health perspectives. 120. 944-51. 10.1289/ehp.1104553.

41. Roberts EM et al., Maternal residence near agricultural pesticide applications and autism spectrum disorders among children in the California Central Valley. Environ Health Perspect. 2007 Oct;115(10):1482-9.

42. Gemmill, A., Gunier, R. B., Bradman, A., Eskenazi, B., & Harley, K. G. (2013). Residential Proximity to Methyl Bromide Use and Birth Outcomes in an Agricultural Population in California. Environmental Health Perspectives, 121(6), 737–743. doi:10.1289/ehp.1205682.

43. https://sustainablepulse.com/2015/10/22/gm-crops-now-banned-in-36-countries-worldwide-sustainable-pulse-research

44. Lerner A, Matthias T. Changes in intestinal tight junction permeability associated with industrial food additives explain the rising incidence of autoimmune disease. Autoimmun Rev, 2015; 14(6):479-489. doi: 10.1016/j.autrev.2015.01.009.

45. Krynytska, Inna & Marushchak, Mariya & Naumova, Lyudmyla & Mazur, Lyudmyla. (2019). The Toxic Impact of Monosodium Glutamate in Rats. Jordan Medical Journal. 53. 91-101.

46. Delahaye F. Should we eat less salt? Arch Cardiovasc Dis 2013;106:324-32.

47. Brown, I.J. & Tzoulaki, Ioanna & Candeias, V. & Elliott, P.. (2009). Salt intakes around the world: Implications for public health international. Int J Epidemiol. 38. 363-384.

48. Ibrahim, Osama. (2018). Sweeteners in Our Diets and World Health Organization Guidelines on Free Sugars Intake. International Journal of Clinical Nutrition & Dietetics. 4. 10.15344/2456-8171/2018/129.

49. Guzmán-Maldonado, H., Paredes-López, O., & Biliaderis, C. G. (1995). Amylolytic enzymes and products derived from starch: A review. Critical Reviews in Food Science and Nutrition, 35(5), 373–403. doi:10.1080/10408399509527706.

50. Airaodion, Augustine & Ogbuagu, Emmanuel & Osemwowa, Etinosa & Ogbuagu, Uloaku & Esonu, Chimdi & Agunbiade, Aanu & Okereke, Davidson & Oloruntoba, Abiodun & Adeniji, Adenike. (2019). Toxicological Effect of Monosodium Glutamate in Seasonings on Human Health. Journal of Food Science and Nutrition. 1. 1-9. 10.33552/GJNFS.2019.01.000522.

51. Yokel, R. A., Hicks, C. L., & Florence, R. L. (2008). Aluminum bioavailability from basic sodium aluminum phosphate, an approved food additive emulsifying agent, incorporated in cheese. Food and Chemical Toxicology, 46(6), 2261–2266. doi:10.1016/j.fct.2008.03.004.

52. Vojdani A. Food immune reactivity and neuroautoimmunity. Funct Neurol Rehabil Ergon, 2014; 4(2-3):175-195.

53. Rao, Meenakshi & Gershon, Michael. (2016). The bowel and beyond: the enteric nervous system in neurological disorders. Nature Reviews Gastroenterology & Hepatology. 13. 10.1038/nrgastro.2016.107.

54. Hirzy, J. & Connett, Paul & Xiang, Q. & Spittle, Bruce & Kennedy, David. (2016). Developmental neurotoxicity of fluoride: A quantitative risk analysis towards establishing a safe daily dose of fluoride for children. 49. 379-400.

55. Strunecka, A.; Patocka, J.; Blaylock, R.L.; Chinoy, N.J. Fluoride interactions: From molecules to disease. Curr. Signal Transd. Ther., 2007, 2, 190-213.

56. Luke, J. Fluoride deposition in the aged human pineal gland. Caries Res., 2001, 35, 125-8.

57. Miodovnik A, Engel SM, Zhu C, Ye X, Soorya LV, Silva MJ et al. Endocrine disruptors and childhood social impairment. Neurotoxicology 2011; 32: 26-1267.

58. Larsson M, Weiss B, Janson S, Sundell J, Bornehag CG. Associations between indoor environmental factors and parental-reported autistic spectrum disorders in children 6-8 years of age. Neurotoxicology 2009; 30: 822--831.

59. Kim, S.M., Han, D.H., Lyoo, H.S., Min, K.J., Kim, K.H., Renshaw, P., 2010. Exposure to environmental toxins in mothers of children with autism spectrum disorder.Psychiatry Investig. 7, 122–127.

60. Testa C, Nuti F, Hayek J, De Felice C, Chelli M, Rovero P et al. Di-(2-ethylhexyl) phthalate and autism spectrum disorders. ASN Neuro 2012; 4: 223-229.

61. Zare Jeddi, Maryam & Janani, Leila & Memari, Amir & Akhondzadeh, Shahin & Yunesian, Masoud. (2016). The role of phthalate esters in autism development: A systematic review. Environmental Research. 151. 10.1016/j.envres.2016.08.021.

62. Stein TP, Schluter MD, Steer RA, Ming X. Autism and phthalate metabolite glucuronidation. J Autism Dev Disord 2013; 43: 2677-2685.

63. Rubin, B.S., 2011. Bisphenol A: an endocrine disruptor with widespread exposure and multiple effects. J. Steroid Biochem. Mol. Biol. 127, 27–34.

64. Kaur, K., Chauhan, V., Gu, F., Chauhan, A., 2014. Bisphenol A induces oxidative stress and mitochondrial dysfunction in lymphoblasts from children with autism and unaffected siblings. Free Radic. Biol. Med. 76, 25–33.

65. Stein TP, Schluter MD, Steer RA, Guo L, Ming X. Bisphenol A exposure in children with autism spectrum disorders. Autism Res 2015; 8(3):272-283.

66. Hertz-Picciotto, Irva & Bergman, Ake & Fängström, Britta & Rose, Melissa & Krakowiak, Paula & Pessah, Isaac & Hansen, Robin & Bennett, Deborah. (2011). Polybrominated diphenyl ethers in relation to autism and developmental delay: A case-control study. Environmental health : a global access science source. 10. 1. 10.1186/1476-069X-10-1.

67. Brent GA. Environmental exposures and autoimmune thyroid disease. Thyroid. 2010;20(7):755-61. doi: 10.1089/thy.2010.1636.

68. https://www.epa.gov/formaldehyde/facts-about-formaldehyde

Chapter Six

1. Buie, T. (2015). Potential Etiologic Factors of Microbiome Disruption in Autism. Clinical Therapeutics, 37(5), 976–983. doi:10.1016/j.clinthera.2015.04.001.
2. Walsh WJ, Isaacson HR, Rehman F, Hall A. 1997. Elevated blood copper/zinc ratios in assaultive young males. Physiol Behav 62:327-329.
3. Kaslow JE (2011) Copper/Zinc Imbalance. Medical Board of California.
4. Faber S, Zinn GM, Kern JC 2nd, et al. The Plasma Zinc/Serum Copper ratio as a biomarker in Children with Autism Spectrum Disorders. Biomarkers 2009; 14:171-180.
5. Vojdani, Aristo & Lambert, Jama & Vojdani, Elroy. (2017). Blood-based markers in autism spectrum disorders Blood-based markers in autism spectrum disorders. Internal Medicine. 3.
6. Vojdani A. Detection of IgE, IgG, IgA and IgM antibodies against raw and processed food antigens. Nutr Metab (Lond) May 2009; 6:22.
7. Vojdani A. The evolution of food immune reactivity testing: Why food IgG or IgA antibody may not be reproducible from one lab to another, and sometimes not even in the same laboratory. Altern Ther Health Med 2015; 21(Suppl 1):8-22.
8. Vojdani A, Kharrazian D, Mukherjee PS. The prevalence of antibodies against wheat and milk proteins in blood donors and their contribution to neuroautoimmune reactivities. Nutrients, 2014; 6(1):15-36, doi:10.3390/nu6010015.
9. Yorbik Ö, Akay C, Sayal A, et al. Zinc status in autistic children. J Trace Elem Exp Med 2004; 17:101-107.
10. Priya MD, Geetha A Level of Trace Elements (Copper, Zinc, Magnesium and Selenium) and Toxic Elements (Lead and Mercury) in the Hair and Nail of Children with Autism. Biol Trace Ele Res 2010:1-11.
11. Blaurock-Busch, E., Amin, O.R., Dessoki, H.H., Rabah, T., 2012. Toxic metals and essential elements in hair and severity of symptoms among children with autism. Maedica 7 (1), 38-48.
12. Adams JB, Holloway CE, George F, et al. Analyses of Toxic Metals and Essential Minerals in the Hair of Arizona Children with Autism and Associated Conditions, and Their Mothers Biological. Trace Ele Res 2006; 110:193-209.
13. Geier, D.A., Kern, J.K., King, P.G., Sykes, L.K., Geier, M.R., 2012. Hair toxic metal concentrations and autism spectrum disorder severity in young children. Int. J. Environ. Res. Public Health 9 (12), 4486-4497.
14. Suzuki T. Hair and Nails: Advantages and Pitfalls when Used in Biological Monitoring. In T. W. Clarkson, L. Friberg, G. F. Nordberg, & P. R.

Sager (Eds.) Biol Monitoring of Toxic Metals. New York: Plenum Press 1988; 623-640.

15. Adams, J.B., Audhya, T., McDonough-Means, S., Rubin, R.A., Quig, D., Geis, E., et al., 2013. Toxicological status of children with autism vs. neurotypical children and the association with autism severity. Biol. Trace Elem. Res. 151 (2), 171-180.

16. Vojdani, Aristo & Lambert, Jama & Vojdani, Elroy. (2017). Association between environmental triggers and neuroautoimmunity in autism spectrum disorders. 3.

17. Mostafa, G. A., and Al-Ayadhi, L. Y. (2012). The relationship between the increased frequency of serum antineuronal antibodies and the severity of autism in children. Eur. J. Paediatr. Neurol. 16, 464-468. doi: 10.1016/j.ejpn.2011.12.010.

18. Mostafa, G. A., and Al-Ayadhi, L. Y. (2012). Reduced serum concentrations of 25-hydroxy vitamin D in children with autism: relation to autoimmunity. J. Neuroinflam. 9:201. doi: 10.1186/1742-2094-9-201.

19. Mostafa, G. A., and Al-Ayadhi, L. Y. (2013). The possible relationship between allergic manifestations and elevated serum levels of brain specific auto-antibodies in autistic children. J. Neuroimmunol. 261, 77-81. doi: 10.1016/j.jneuroim.2013.04.003.

Chapter Seven

1. Adams, James & Audhya, Tapan & Geis, Elizabeth & Gehn, Eva & Fimbres, Valeria & Pollard, Elena & Mitchell, Jessica & Ingram, Julie & Hellmers, Robert & Laake, Dana & Matthews, Julie & Li, Kefeng & Naviaux, Jane & Naviaux, Robert & Adams, Rebecca & Coleman, Devon & Quig, David. (2018). Comprehensive Nutritional and Dietary Intervention for Autism Spectrum Disorder--A Randomized, Controlled 12-Month Trial. Nutrients. 10. 369. 10.3390/nu10030369.

2. Millward, C.; Ferriter, M.; Calver, S.; Connell-Jones, G. Gluten- and casein-free diets for autistic spectrum disorder. Cochrane Database Syst. Rev. 2008, 2, CD003498.

3. Whiteley, P.; Haracopos, D.; Knivsberg, A.M.; Reichelt, K.L.; Parlar, S.; Jacobsen, J.; Seim, A.; Pedersen, L.; Schondel, M.; Shattock, P. The ScanBrit randomised, controlled, single-blind study of a gluten- and casein-free dietary intervention for children with autism spectrum disorders. Nutr. Neurosci. 2010, 13, 87–100.

4. deMagistris L, Picardi A, Siniscalco D, Riccio MP, Sapone A, Cariello R, Abbadessa S, Medici N, Lammers KM, Schiraldi C, Iardino P, Marotta R, Tolone C, Fasano A, Pascotto A, Bravaccio C. Antibodies against food antigens in patients with autistic spectrum disorders (ASDs). Biomed Res Int. 2013;. doi:10.1155/2013/729349.

REFERENCES

5. Mezzelani A, Landini M, Facchiano F, Raggi ME, Villa L, Molteni M, et al. Environment, dysbiosis, immunity and sex-specific susceptibility: a translational hypothesis for regressive autism pathogenesis. Nutr Neurosci 2015;18(4):14561. doi:10.1179/1476830513Y.0000000108.

6. Whiteley P, Shattock P, Knivsberg A-M, et al. Gluten- and casein-free dietary intervention for autism spectrum conditions. Front Hum Neurosci, Jan 2012; 6:344.

7. Pennesi CM, Klein LC (2012) Effectiveness of the gluten-free, casein-free diet for children diagnosed with autism spectrum disorder: based on parental report. Nutr Neurosci 15:85-91.

8. de Magistris L, Familiari V, Pascotto A, Sapone A, Frolli A, Iardino P, et al. Alterations of the intestinal barrier in patients with autism spectrum disorders and in their first-degree relatives. J Pediatr Gastroenterol Nutr. (2010) 51:418–24. doi: 10.1097/MPG.0b013e3181dcc4a5.

9. A. Vojdani, T. O'Bryan, J. A. Green et al., "Immune response to dietary proteins, gliadin and cerebellar peptides in children with autism," Nutritional Neuroscience, vol. 7, no. 3, pp. 151-161, 2004.

10. H. Jyonouchi, S. Sun, and N. Itokazu, "Innate immunity associated with inflammatory responses and cytokine production against common dietary proteins in patients with autism spectrum disorder," Neuropsychobiology, vol. 46, no. 2, pp. 76-84, 2002.

11. Fasano A, Sapone A, Zevallos V, Schuppan D, Non-celiac Gluten Sensitivity, Gastroenterology (2015), doi: 10.1053/j.gastro.2014.12.049.

12. Catassi C, Bai JC, Bonaz B, et al. Non-celiac gluten sensitivity: the new frontier of gluten related disorders. Nutrients. 2013;5(10):3839-3853.

13. Lerner A, Matthias T. Changes in intestinal tight junction permeability associated with industrial food additives explain the rising incidence of autoimmune disease. Autoimmun Rev, 2015; 14(6):479-489. doi: 10.1016/j.autrev.2015.01.009.

14. Vojdani, Aristo & Lambert, Jama & Vojdani, Elroy. (2017). Blood-based markers in autism spectrum disorders Blood-based markers in autism spectrum disorders. Internal Medicine. 3.

15. Vojdani, Aristo & Lambert, Jama & Vojdani, Elroy. (2017). Association between environmental triggers and neuroautoimmunity in autism spectrum disorders. 3.

16. Vojdani A. Food immune reactivity and neuroautoimmunity. Funct Neurol Rehabil Ergon, 2014; 4(2-3):175-195.

17. Jyonouchi, H., Geng, L., Ruby, A., Reddy, C., Zimmerman-Bier, B., 2005. Evaluation of an association between gastrointestinal symptoms and cytokine production against common dietary proteins in children with autism spectrum disorders. J. Pediatr. 146, 605-610.

18. Reichelt, K.L., Ekrem, J. and Scott, H. (1990) "Gluten, milk proteins and autism: dietary intervention effects on behavior and peptide secretion", J. Appl. Nutr. 42, 111.

19. Shattock, P., Kennedy, A., Rowell, F. and Berney, T. (1991) "Role of neuropeptides in autism and their relationship with classical neurotransmitters", Brain Dysfunct. 3, 328-345.

20. Reichelt, K.L. (1994) "Biochemistry and psychophysiology of autistic syndromes", Tidsskr. Nor. Laegeforen. 114, 1432-1434.

21. Reichelt, W.H. and Reichelt, K.L. (1997) "The possible role of peptides derived from food proteins in diseases of the nervous system", In: Gobbi, G., ed, Epilepsy and other Neurological Disorders in Coeliac Disease (John Libbey & Co., London), pp 225-235.

22. Whiteley, P., Rodgers, J., Savery, D. and Shattock, P. (1999) "A gluten-free diet as an intervention for autism and associated spectrum disorders: preliminary findings", Autism3, 45-65.

23. Horvath, K., Papadimitriou, J.C., Rabsztyn, A., Drachenberg, C. and Tildon, J.T. (1999) "Gastrointestinal abnormalities in children with autistic disorder", J. Pediatr. 135, 559-563.

24. Nelson, K.B., Grether, J.K., Croen, L.A., Dambrosia, J.M., Dickens, B.F., Jeliffe, L.L., Hansen, R.L. and Phillips, T.M. (2001) "Neuropeptides and neurotrophins in neonatal blood of children with autism and mental retardation", Ann. Neurol. 49, 597-606.

25. Reichelt, K.L. and Knivsberg, A.M. (2003) "Can the pathophysiology of autism be explained by the nature of the discovered urine peptides?", Nutr. Neurosci. 6, 19-28.

26. Cazzullo, Adriana & Musetti, Maria & Musetti, Laura & Bajo, Sonia & Sacerdote, Paola & Panerai, Alberto. (1999). β-Endorphin levels in peripheral blood mononuclear cells and long-term naltrexone treatment in autistic children. European neuropsychopharmacology : the journal of the European College of Neuropsychopharmacology. 9. 361-6. 10.1016/S0924-977X(99)00010-3.

27. Sokolov O, Kost N, Andreeva O, Korneeva E, Meshavkin V, Tarakanova Y, et al. Autistic children display elevated urine levels of bovine casomorphin-7 immunoreactivity. Peptides 2014;56:68-71.

28. Tordjman S, Anderson GM, Botbol M, Brailly-Tabard S, Perez-Diaz F, Graignic R, et al. Pain reactivity and plasma beta-endorphin in children and adolescents with autistic disorder. PLoS ONE 2009;4(8):e5289.

29. Cieślińska, A., Sienkiewicz-Szłapka, E., Wasilewska, J., Fiedorowicz, E., Chwała, B., Moszyńska-Dumara, M., ... Kostyra, E. (2015). Influence of candidate polymorphisms on the dipeptidyl peptidase IV and μ-opioid receptor genes expression in aspect of the β-casomorphin-7 modulation functions in autism. Peptides, 65, 6–11. doi:10.1016/j.peptides.2014.11.012.

30. Shah JJ, Trivedi M, Hodgson N, Deth R. Casein and gluten-derived opiate peptides affect cysteine uptake and redox status. FASEB J 2013;27:107581.

31. Sokolov O, Kost N, Andreeva O, Korneeva E, Meshavkin V, Tarakanova Y,et al. Autistic children display elevated urine levels of bovine casomorphin-7immunoreactivity. Peptides 2014;56:68-71.

32. Wasilewska J, Sienkiewicz-Szłapka E, Ku´zbida E, Jarmołowska B, KaczmarskiM, Kostyra E. The exogenous opioid peptides and DPPIV serum activity in infants with apnoea expressed as apparent life threatening events (ALTE). Neu-ropeptides 2011;45:189–95.

33. Kaczmarski, Maciej & Wasilewska, Jolanta & Lasota, M. (2005). Hypersensitivity to hydrolyzed cow's milk protein formula in infants and young

children with atopic eczema/dermatitis syndrome with cow's milk protein allergy. Roczniki Akademii Medycznej w Białymstoku (1995). 50. 274-8.

34. Whiteley P, Shattock P. Biochemical aspects in autism spectrum disorders:updating the opioid-excess theory and presenting new opportunities for biomedical intervention. Expert Opin Ther Targets 2002;6(2):175–83.

35. Hunter LC, O'Hare A, Herron WJ, Fisher LA, Jones GE. Opioid peptides and dipeptidyl peptidase in autism. Dev Med Child Neurol 2003;45(2):121–8.

36. Wasilewska J, Jarocka-Cyrta E, Kaczmarski M. The pathogenesis of gastroin-testinal disorders in children with autism. Pol Merkur Lek 2009;27:40–3.

37. Jyonouchi, H., Sun, S.N. and Le, H. (2001) "Proinflammatory and regulatory cytokine production associated with innate and adaptive immune responses in children with autism spectrum disorders and developmental regression", J. Neuroimmunol. 120, 170-179.

38. Knivsberg, A.M., Reichelt, K.L., Nødland, M. and Høein, T. (1995) "Autistic syndromes and diet: a follow up study", Scand. J. Edu. Res. 39, 223-236.

39. Knivsberg, A.M., Reichelt, K.L. and Nødland, M. (2001) "Reports on dietary intervention in autistic disorders", Nutr. Neurosci. 4, 25-37.

40. Knivsberg AM, Reichelt KL, Hoien T, Nodland M. A randomised, controlled study of dietary intervention in autistic syndromes. Nutr Neurosci. 2002;5(4):251-261.

41. Goyer RA Toxic and Essential Metal Interactions. Ann Rev of Nutr 1997; 17: 37-50.

42. Goyer, R. A. (1995). Nutrition and metal toxicity. The American Journal of Clinical Nutrition, 61(3), 646S–650S. doi:10.1093/ajcn/61.3.646s.

43. Napoli, Eleonora & Duenas, Nadia & Giulivi, Cecilia. (2014). Potential Therapeutic Use of the Ketogenic Diet in Autism Spectrum Disorders. Frontiers in pediatrics. 2. 69. 10.3389/fped.2014.00069.

44. Evangeliou A, Vlachonikolis I, Mihailidou H, Spilioti M, Skarpalezou A, Makaronas N, et al. Application of a ketogenic diet in children with autistic behavior: pilot study. J Child Neurol (2003) 18:113-8. doi:10.1177/08830738030180020501.

45. Herbert MR, Buckley JA. Autism and dietary therapy: case report and review of the literature. J Child Neurol (2013) 28:975-82. doi:10.1177/0883073813488668.

Chapter Eight

1. Rossignol DA, Genuis SJ, Frye RE. Environmental toxicants and autism spectrum disorders: a systematic review. Transl Psychiatry, Feb 2014; 4:e360.

2. Lu, C., Toepel, K., Irish, R., Fenske, R. A., Barr, D. B., & Bravo, R. (2006). Organic Diets Significantly Lower Children's Dietary Exposure to Organophosphorus Pesticides. Environmental Health Perspectives, 114(2), 260–263. doi:10.1289/ehp.8418.

3. Bradman, A., Quirós-Alcalá, L., Castorina, R., Schall, R. A., Camacho, J., Holland, N. T., ... Eskenazi, B. (2015). Effect of Organic Diet Intervention on Pesticide Exposures in Young Children Living in Low-Income Urban and Agricultural Communities. Environmental Health Perspectives, 123(10), 1086–1093. doi:10.1289/ehp.1408660.

4. Barański, M., Średnicka-Tober, D., Volakakis, N., Seal, C., Sanderson, R., Stewart, G. B., ... Leifert, C. (2014). Higher antioxidant and lower cadmium concentrations and lower incidence of pesticide residues in organically grown crops: a systematic literature review and meta-analyses. British Journal of Nutrition, 112(05), 794–811. doi:10.1017/s0007114514001366.

5. Yang Q. Gain weight by "going diet?" Artificial sweeteners and the neurobiology of sugar cravings: Neuroscience 2010. Yale J Biol Med. 2010;83(2):101–108.

6. https://ntp.niehs.nih.gov/ntp/roc/content/profiles/butylatedhydroxyanisole.pdf

7. McCann et al, Food additives and hyperactive behaviour in 3-year-old and 8/9-year-old children in the community: a randomised, double-blinded, placebo-controlled trial. Lancet. 2007 Nov 3;370(9598):1560-7. Erratum in: Lancet. 2007 Nov 3;370(9598):1542.

Chapter Nine

1. Klukowski M, Wasilewska J, Lebensztejn D. Sleep and gastrointestinal disturbances in autism spectrum disorder in children. Dev Period Med. 2015;19(2):157–61.

2. Engelhardt CR, Mazurek MO, Sohl K. Media use and sleep among boys with autism spectrum disorder, ADHD, or typical development. Pediatrics, 2013;132:1081-1089.

3. Krakowiak P, Goodlin-Jones B, Hertz-Picciotto I, Croen LA, Hansen RL. Sleep problems in children with autism spectrum disorders, developmental delays, and typical development: A population-based study. J Sleep Res, 2008;17:197-206.

4. Rossignol DA, Frye RE. Melatonin in autism spectrum disorders. Curr Clin Pharmacol. 2014;9(4):326-34.

5. Rossignol DA, Frye RE. Melatonin in autism spectrum disorders: a systematic review and meta-analysis. Dev Med Child Neurol. 2011;53(9):783-92.

6. Liu X, Hubbard JA, Fabes RA, Adam JB. Sleep disturbances and correlates of children with autism spectrum disorders. Child Psychiatry Hum Dev, 2006;37:179-191.

7. Xie, Lulu & Kang, Hongyi & Xu, Qiwu & Chen, Michael & Liao, Yong-hong & Thiyagarajan, Meenakshisundaram & O'Donnell, John & Christensen, Daniel & Nicholson, Charles & Iliff, Jeffrey & Takano, Takahiro & Deane, Rashid & Nedergaard, Maiken. (2013). Sleep Drives Metabolite Clearance from the Adult Brain. Science (New York, N.Y.). 342. 373-7. 10.1126/science.1241224.

8. Turner TH, Drummond SP, Salamat JS, Brown GG. Effects of 42 hr of total sleep deprivation on component processes of verbal working memory. Neuropsychology, 2007;21:787-795.

9. Johnson CR, Turner KS, Foldes E, Brooks MM, Kronk R, Wiggs L. Behavioral parent training to address sleep disturbances in young children with autism spectrum disorder: A pilot trial. Sleep Med, 2013;14:995-1004.

10. Nadeau JM, Arnold EB, Keene AC, et al. Frequency and clinical correlates of sleep-related problems among anxious youth with autism spectrum disorders. Child Psychiatry Hum Dev. 2015;46(4):558–66.

11. Hill AP, Zuckerman KE, Hagen AD, et al. Aggressive behavior problems in children with autism spectrum disorders: prevalence and correlates in a large clinical sample. Res Autism Spectr Disord. 2014;8(9):1121–33.

12. Schreck KA, Mulick JA, Smith AF. Sleep problems as possible predictors of intensifed symptoms of autism. Res Dev Disabil, 2004;25:57-66.

13. Maquet P. The role of sleep in learning and memory. Science. 2001;294(5544):1048-1052.

14. Sikora DM, Johnson K, Clemons T, Katz T. The relationship between sleep problems and daytime behavior in children of different ages with autism spectrum disorders. Pediatrics 2012; 130 (Suppl 2):S83-S90.

15. Taylor MA, Schreck KA, Mulick JA. Sleep disruption as a correlate to cognitive and adaptive behavior problems in autism spectrum disorders. Res Dev Disabil 2012; 33:1408-1417.

16. Malow, Beth & Adkins, Karen & McGrew, Susan & Wang, Lily & Goldman, Suzanne & Fawkes, Diane & Burnette, Courtney. (2011). Melatonin for Sleep in Children with Autism: A Controlled Trial Examining Dose, Tolerability, and Outcomes. Journal of autism and developmental disorders. 42. 1729-37; author reply 1738. 10.1007/s10803-011-1418-3.

17. Tilford JM, Payakachat N, Kuhlthau KA, et al. Treatment for sleep problems in children with autism and caregiver spillover effects. J Autism Dev Disord. 2015;45(11):3613–23.

18. Doo S, Wing YK. Sleep problems of children with pervasive developmental disorders: Correlation with parental stress. Dev Med Child Neurol, 2006;48:650-655.

19. Patzold LM, Richdale AL, Tonge BJ. An investigation into sleep characteristics of children with autism and Asperger's disorder. J Paediatr Child Health, 1998;34:528-533.

20. Richdale, A., Frances, A., Gavidia-Payne, S., & Cotton, S. (2000). Parental stress, behaviour, and sleep problems in children with an intellectual disability. Journal of Intellectual and Developmental Disability, 5, 47-161.

21. Goldman, S. E., Richdale, A. L., Clemons, T., & Malow, B. A. (2012). Parental sleep concerns in autism spectrum disorders: Variations from childhood to adolescence. Journal of Autism and Developmental Disorders, 42(4), 531-538.

22. Kuhn, J. C., & Carter, A. S. (2006). Maternal self-efficacy and associated parenting cognitions among mothers of children with autism. American Journal of Orthopsychiatry, 76(4), 564-575.

23. Horvath K, Perman JA. Autism and gastrointestinal symptoms. Curr Gastroenterol Rep, 2002;4:251-258.

24. Molloy CA, Manning-Courtney P. Prevalence of chronic gastrointestinal symptoms in children with autism and autistic spectrum disorders. Autism, 2003;7:165-171.

25. Valicenti-McDermott M, McVicar K, Rapin I, Wershil BK, Cohen H, Shinnar S. Frequency of gastrointestinal symptoms in children with autistic spectrum disorders and association with family history of autoimmune disease. J Dev Behav Pediatr, 2006;27:S128-S136.

26. Liu X, Hubbard JA, Fabes RA, Adam JB. Sleep disturbances and correlates of children with autism spectrum disorders. Child Psychiatry Hum Dev, 2006;37:179-191.

27. Bubenik, G.A., 2002. Gastrointestinal melatonin: localization, function, and clinical relevance. Dig. Dis. Sci. 47, 2336-2348.

28. Sivertsen B, Posserud MB, Gillberg C, et al. Sleep problems in children with autism spectrum problems: a longitudinal population-based study. Autism 2012; 16:139-150.

29. Malow BA, Adkins KW, Reynolds A, Weiss SK, Loh A, Fawkes D, Katz T, Goldman SE, Madduri N, Hundley R, Clemons T. Parent-based sleep education for children with autism spectrum disorders. J Autism Dev Disord, 2014;44:216-228.

30. Revell, V.L., Skene, D.J., 2007. Light-induced melatonin suppression in humans with polychromatic and monochromatic light. Chronobiol. Int. 24, 1125-1135.

31. Melke J, Goubran Botros H, Chaste P, et al. Abnormal melatonin synthesis in autism spectrum disorders. Mol Psychiatry. 2008; 13(1):90-98.

32. Nir I, Meir D, Zilber N, Knobler H, Hadjez J, Lerner Y. Brief report: circadian melatonin, thyroid-stimulating hormone, prolactin, and cortisol levels in serum of young adults with autism. J Autism Dev Disord. 1995;25(6):641-654.

33. Tordjman S, Anderson GM, Pichard N, Charbuy H, Touitou Y. Nocturnal excretion of 6-sulphatoxymelatonin in children and adolescents with autistic disorder. Biol Psychiatry. 2005;57(2):134-138.

34. Tordjman S, Anderson GM, Bellissant E, et al. Day and nighttime excretion of 6-sulphatoxymelatonin in adolescents and young adults with autistic disorder. Psychoneuroendocrinology 2012; 37:1990-1997.

35. Rossignol DA, Frye RE. Melatonin in autism spectrum disorders: a systematic review and meta-analysis. Dev Med Child Neurol 2011; 53:783-792.

36. Leu RM, Beyderman L, Botzolakis EJ, et al. Relation of melatonin to sleep architecture in children with autism. J Autism Dev Disord 2011; 41:427-433.

Chapter Ten

1.   Adams, James & Audhya, Tapan & Geis, Elizabeth & Gehn, Eva & Fimbres, Valeria & Pollard, Elena & Mitchell, Jessica & Ingram, Julie & Hellmers, Robert & Laake, Dana & Matthews, Julie & Li, Kefeng & Naviaux, Jane & Naviaux, Robert & Adams, Rebecca & Coleman, Devon & Quig, David. (2018). Comprehensive Nutritional and Dietary Intervention for Autism Spectrum Disorder--A Randomized, Controlled 12-Month Trial. Nutrients. 10. 369. 10.3390/nu10030369.

2.   Adams, James & Audhya, Tapan & McDonough-Means, Sharon & Rubin, Robert & Quig, David & Geis, Elizabeth & Gehn, Eva & Loresto, Melissa & Mitchell, Jessica & Atwood, Sharon & Barnhouse, Suzanne & Lee, Wondra. (2011). Effect of a vitamin/mineral supplement on children and adults with autism. BMC pediatrics. 11. 111. 10.1186/1471-2431-11-111.

3.   Mehl-Madrona L et al., Micronutrients versus standard medication management in autism: a naturalistic case-control study. J Child Adolesc Psychopharmacol 2010, 20(2):95-103.

4.   Horvath, Karoly & Papadimitriou, John & Rabsztyn, Anna & Drachenberg, Cinthia & Tildon, J.Tyson. (1999). Gastrointestinal abnormalities in children with autistic disorder. The Journal of pediatrics. 135. 559-63. 10.1016/S0022-3476(99)70052-1.

5.   Williams, Brent & Hornig, Mady & Buie, Timothy & Bauman, Margaret & Paik, Myunghee & Wick, Ivan & Bennett, Ashlee & Jabado, Omar & Hirschberg, David & Lipkin, W. (2011). Impaired carbohydrate digestion and transport and mucosal dysbiosis in the intestines of children with autism and gastrointestinal disturbances. PloS one. 6. e24585. 10.1371/journal.pone.0024585.

6.   Kushak, Rafail & Lauwers, Gregory & Winter, Harland & Buie, Timothy. (2011). Intestinal disaccharidase activity in patients with autism: Effect of age, gender, and intestinal inflammation. Autism : the international journal of research and practice. 15. 285-94. 10.1177/1362361310369142.

7.   Brudnak MA, Rimland B, Kerry RE, Dailey M, Taylor R, Stayton B, et al. Enzyme-based therapy for autism spectrum disorders is it worth another look? Med Hypotheses (2002) 58:422-8. doi: 10.1054/mehy.2001.1513.

8.   Saad K, Eltayeb AA, Mohamad IL, Al-Atram AA, Elserogy Y, Bjorklund G, et al. A randomized, placebo-controlled trial of digestive enzymes in children with autism spectrum disorders. Clin Psychopharmacol Neurosci. (2015) 13:18893. doi: 10.9758/cpn.2015.13.2.188.

9.   Sanctuary, M.R.; Kain, J.N.; Chen, S.Y.; Kalanetra, K.; Lemay, D.G.; Rose, D.R.; Yang, H.T.; Tancredi, D.J.; German, J.B.; Slupsky, C.M.; et al. Pilot study of probiotic/colostrum supplementation on gut function in children with autism and gastrointestinal symptoms. PLoS ONE 2019, 14, e0210064.

10. Kaluzna-Czaplinska J, Blaszczyk S. The level of arabinitol in autistic children after probiotic therapy. Nutrition (2012) 28:1246.doi: 10.1016/j.nut.2011.08.002.

11. Parracho, H.M.; Gibson, G.R.; Knott, F.; Bosscher, D.; Kleerebezem, M.; McCartney, A.L. A double-blind, placebo-controlled, crossover-designed probiotic feeding study in children diagnosed with autistic spectrum disorders. Int. J. Probiotics Prebiotics 2010, 5, 69-74.

12. Shaaban, S.Y.; El Gendy, Y.G.; Mehanna, N.S.; El-Senousy, W.M.; El-Feki, H.S.; Saad, K.; El-Asheer, O.M. The role of probiotics in children with autism spectrum disorder: A prospective, open-label study. Nutr. Neurosci. 2018, 21, 676-681.

13. West, R.; Roberts, E.; Sichel, L.S.; Sichel, J. Improvements in gastrointestinal symptoms among children with autism spectrum disorder receiving the Delpro® Probiotic and immunomodulator formulation. J. Prob. Health 2013, 1, 102.

14. Doenyas, Ceymi. (2018). Gut Microbiota, Inflammation, and Probiotics on Neural Development in Autism Spectrum Disorder. Neuroscience. 374. 271-286. 10.1016/j.neuroscience.2018.01.060.

15. Patrick L and Salik R, The Effect of Essential Fatty Acid Supplementation on Language Development and Learning Skills in Autism and Asperger's syndrome. Autism/Asperger's Digest: Research Article – Jan/Feb 2005.

16. Meguid et al, Role of polyunsaturated fatty acids in the management of Egyptian children with autism. Clinical Biochemistry 41 (2008) 1044-1048.

17. Bell JG et al, The fatty acid compositions of erythrocyte and plasma polar lipids in children with autism, developmental delay or typically developing controls and the effect of fish oil intake. Br J Nutr. 2010 Apr;103(8):1160-7.

18. Bent et al.,. Effects of large doses of arachidonic acid added to docosahexaenoic acid on social impairment in individuals with autism spectrum disorders: a double-blind, placebo-controlled, randomized trial. J Clin Psychopharmacol. 2012 Apr;32(2):200-6.

19. Mazahery, H.; Stonehouse, W.; Delshad, M.; Kruger, M.C.; Conlon, C.A.; Beck, K.L.; von Hurst, P.R. Relationship between Long Chain n-3 Polyunsaturated Fatty Acids and Autism Spectrum Disorder: Systematic Review and Meta-Analysis of Case-Control and Randomised Controlled Trials. Nutrients 2017, 9, 155.

20. Goyer RA Toxic and Essential Metal Interactions. Ann Rev of Nutr 1997; 17: 37-50.

21. Goyer, R. A. (1995). Nutrition and metal toxicity. The American Journal of Clinical Nutrition, 61(3), 646S–650S. doi:10.1093/ajcn/61.3.646s.

22. Blaylock, R.L. Excitotoxicity, a possible central mechanism in fluoride neurotoxicity. Fluoride, 2004, 37, 264-77.

Chapter Eleven

1. James SJ, Cutler et al., Metabolic biomarkers of increased oxidative stress and impaired methylation capacity in children with autism. Am J Clin Nutr. 2004, 80(6):1611-7.

2. James SJ, Melnyk S, Fuchs G, Reid T, Jernigan S, Pavliv O, Hubanks A, Gaylor DW: Efficacy of methylcobalamin and folinic acid treatment on glutathione redox status in children with autism. Am J Clin Nutr 2009, 89(1):425-30.

3. S. J. James, S. Melnyk, G. Fuchs et al., "Efficacy of methylcobalamin and folinic acid treatment on glutathione redox status in children with autism," American Journal of Clinical Nutrition, vol. 89, no. 1, pp. 425-430, 2009.

4. Frye R, Slattery J, Delhey L, Furgerson B, Strickland T, Tippett M, et al. Folinic acid improves verbal communication in children with autism and language impairment: a randomized double-blind placebo-controlled trial. Mol Psychiatry (2016). doi:10.1038/mp.2016.168.

5. Bertoglio K, Jill James S, Deprey L, Brule N, Hendren RL. Pilot study of the effect of methyl B12 treatment on behavioral and biomarker measures in children with autism. J Altern Complement Med (2010) 16(5):555-60. doi:10.1089/acm.2009.0177.

6. Hendren RL, James SJ, Widjaja F, Lawton B, Rosenblatt A, Bent S. Randomized, placebo-controlled trial of methyl B12 for children with autism. J Child Adolesc Psychopharmacol (2016) 26(9):774-83. doi:10.1089/cap.2015.0159.

7. Frye RE, Melnyk S, Fuchs G, Reid T, Jernigan S, Pavliv O, et al. Effectiveness of methylcobalamin and folinic acid treatment on adaptive behavior in children with autistic disorder is related to glutathione redox status. Autism Res Treat 2013; 2013: 609-705.

8. Adams, James & Audhya, Tapan & McDonough-Means, Sharon & Rubin, Robert & Quig, David & Geis, Elizabeth & Gehn, Eva & Loresto, Melissa & Mitchell, Jessica & Atwood, Sharon & Barnhouse, Suzanne & Lee, Wondra. (2011). Nutritional and Metabolic Status of Children with Autism vs. Neurotypical Children, and the Association with Autism Severity. Nutrition & metabolism. 8. 34. 10.1186/1743-7075-8-34.

9. Adams JB, George F, Audhya T: Abnormally high plasma levels of vitamin B6 in children with autism not taking supplements compared to controls not taking supplements. J Altern Complement Med 2006, 12(1):59-63.

10. Saad, K.; Abdel-Rahman, A.A.; Elserogy, Y.M.; Al-Atram, A.A.; Cannell, J.J.; Bjorklund, G.; Abdel-Reheim, M.K.; Othman, H.A.; El-Houfey, A.A.; Abd El-Aziz, N.H.; et al. Vitamin D status in Autism Spectrum Disorders and the efficacy of vitamin D supplementation in autistic children. Nutr. Neurosci. 2015.

11. Feng, J.; Shan, L.; Du, L.; Wang, B.; Li, H.; Wang, W.; Wang, T.; Dong, H.; Yue, X.; Xu, Z.; et al. Clinical improvement following vitamin D3 supplementation in Autism Spectrum Disorder. Nutr. Neurosci. 2016.

12. Meguid, N. A., Bjørklund, G., Gebril, O. H., Doşa, M. D., Anwar, M., Elsaeid, A., ... Chirumbolo, S. (2019). The role of zinc supplementation on the metallothionein system in children with autism spectrum disorder. Acta Neurologica Belgica. doi:10.1007/s13760-019-01181-9.

13. Russo AJ, de Vito R (2011) Analysis of copper and zinc plasma concentration the efficacy of zinc therapy in individuals with Asperger's syndrome,

pervasive developmental disorder not otherwise specified (PDD-NOS) and autism. Biomark Insights 6:127–133.

14. Russo AJ. Increased Copper in Individuals with Autism Normalizes Post Zinc Therapy More Efficiently in Individuals with Concurrent GI Disease. Nutrition and Metabolic Insights 2011;4: 49-54.

15. Osredkar J, Sustar N (2011) Copper and Zinc, Biological Role and Significance of Copper/Zinc Imbalance. J Clinic Toxicol S3:001. doi:10.4172/2161-0494.S3-001.

16. Blaurock-Busch, E., Amin, O.R., Dessoki, H.H., Rabah, T., 2012. Toxic metals and essential elements in hair and severity of symptoms among children with autism. Maedica 7 (1), 38-48.

17. Priya MD, Geetha A Level of Trace Elements (Copper, Zinc, Magnesium and Selenium) and Toxic Elements (Lead and Mercury) in the Hair and Nail of Children with Autism. Biol Trace Ele Res 2010:1-11.

18. Jory J, Woody R Red-Cell Trace Minerals in Children with Autism McGinnis. Am J Biochem Biotech 2008; 4:101-104

19. Watts DL (1994) The nutritional relationships of selenium. J Orthomol Med 9:111-117.

20. Adams, James & Audhya, Tapan & Geis, Elizabeth & Gehn, Eva & Fimbres, Valeria & Pollard, Elena & Mitchell, Jessica & Ingram, Julie & Hellmers, Robert & Laake, Dana & Matthews, Julie & Li, Kefeng & Naviaux, Jane & Naviaux, Robert & Adams, Rebecca & Coleman, Devon & Quig, David. (2018). Comprehensive Nutritional and Dietary Intervention for Autism Spectrum Disorder--A Randomized, Controlled 12-Month Trial. Nutrients. 10. 369. 10.3390/nu10030369.

21. Waring RH, Ngong JM, Klovsra L, Green S, Sharp H: Biochemical Parameters in Autistic Children. Dev Brain Dysfunct 1997, 10:40-43.

22. Geier DA, Kern JK, Garver CR, Adams JB, Audhya T, Geier MR: A prospective study of transsulfuration biomarkers in autistic disorders. Neurochem Res 2009, 34(2):386-93, Erratum in: Neurochem Res. 2009, 34(2):394.

23. O'Reilly, B.A.; Warning, R.H. Enzyme and Sulphur Oxidation Deficiencies in Autistic Children with Known Food/Chemical Sensitivities. J. Orthomol. Med. 1993, 8, 198–200.

24. Alberti, A.; Pirrone, P.; Elia, M.;Waring, R.H.; Romano, C. Sulphation deficit in "low-functioning" autistic children: A pilot study. Biol. Psychiatry 1999, 46, 420–424.

25. Horvath, K.; Perman, J.A. Autistic disorder and gastrointestinal disease. Curr. Opin. Pediatr. 2002, 14, 583–587.

26. Schrauzer, G. N., Shrestha, K. P., & Flores-Arce, M. F. (1992). Lithium in scalp hair of adults, students, and violent criminals. Biological Trace Element Research, 34(2), 161–176. doi:10.1007/bf02785244.

27. Adams JB, Holloway CE, George F, Quig D: Analyses of toxic metals and essential minerals in the hair of Arizona children with autism and associated conditions, and their mothers. Biol Trace Elem Res 2006, 110(3):193-209.

28. Deepmala, Slattery J, Kumar N, et al. Clinical trials of N-acetylcysteine in psychiatry and neurology: a systematic review. Neurosci Biobehav Rev. 2015;55:294-321.

29. Hardan AY, Fung LK, Libove RA, et al. A randomized controlled pilot trial of oral N-acetylcysteine in children with autism. Biol Psychiatry. 2012;71(11):956–61.

30. Ghanizadeh A, Moghimi-Sarani E. A randomized double blind placebo controlled clinical trial of N-Acetylcysteine added to risperidone for treating autistic disorders. BMC Psychiatry. 2013;13(1):196.

31. Dean O, Giorlando F, Berk M. N-acetylcysteine in psychiatry: current therapeutic evidence and potential mechanisms of action. J Psychiatry Neurosci 2011;36:78-86.

32. Dinicola, Simona & Grazia, S & Carlomagno, Gianfranco & Pintucci, J. (2014). N-acetylcysteine as powerful molecule to destroy bacterial biofilms. A systematic review. European review for medical and pharmacological sciences. 18. 2942-8.

33. Samuni, Yuval & Goldstein, Sara & Dean, Olivia & Berk, Michael. (2013). The chemistry and biological activities of N-acetylcysteine. Biochimica et biophysica acta. 1830. 10.1016/j.bbagen.2013.04.016.

34. INAGAWA, Kentaro & HIRAOKA, Takenori & KOHDA, Tohru & Yamadera, Wataru & Takahashi, Michio. (2006). Subjective effects of glycine ingestion before bedtime on sleep quality. Sleep and Biological Rhythms. 4. 75 - 77. 10.1111/j.1479-8425.2006.00193.x.

35. Yamadera, Wataru & INAGAWA, Kentaro & Chiba, Shintaro & Bannai, Makoto & Takahashi, Michio & NAKAYAMA, Kazuhiko. (2007). Glycine ingestion improves subjective sleep quality in human volunteers, correlating with polysomnographic changes. Sleep and Biological Rhythms. 5. 126 - 131. 10.1111/j.1479-8425.2007.00262.x.

36. Bannai, Makoto & Kawai, Nobuhiro & Ono, Kaori & Nakahara, Keiko & Murakami, Noboru. (2012). The Effects of Glycine on Subjective Daytime Performance in Partially Sleep-Restricted Healthy Volunteers. Frontiers in neurology. 3. 61. 10.3389/fneur.2012.00061.

37. Saransaari P, Oja SS (2000) Taurine and neural cell damage. Amino Acids 19: 509-526.

38. Kern, J.K., Geier, D.A., Adams, J.B., Garver, C.R., Audhya, T., & Geier, M.R. (2011). A clinical trial of glutathione supplementation in autism spectrum disorders. Medical Science Monitor: International Medical Journal of Experimental and Clinical Research, 17, CR677-CR682.

39. Tu, W.J., Chen, H., & He, J. (2012). Application of LC-MS/MS analysis of plasma amino acids profiles in children with autism. Journal of Clinical Biochemistry and Nutrition, 51, 248249. http://doi.org/10.3164/jcbn.12-45.

40. Ming X, Stein TP, Barnes V, Rhodes N, Guo L. Metabolic perturbance in autism spectrum disorders: a metabolomics study. J Proteome 2012;11:585662.

41. Chez MG, Buchanan CP, Aimonovitch MC, et al. Double-blind, placebo-controlled study of L-carnosine supplementation in children with autistic spectrum disorders. J Child Neurol. 2002;17(11):833–7.

42. Hajizadeh-Zaker, R., Ghajar, A., Mesgarpour, B., Afarideh, M., Mohammadi, M.-R., & Akhondzadeh, S. (2018). l-Carnosine As an Adjunctive

Therapy to Risperidone in Children with Autistic Disorder: A Randomized, Double-Blind, Placebo-Controlled Trial. Journal of Child and Adolescent Psychopharmacology, 28(1), 74–81. doi:10.1089/cap.2017.0026.

43. Hipkiss, Alan. (2018). Energy metabolism and autism: the ameliorative potential of carnosine and agmatine. Neurological Disorders and Therapeutics. 2. 10.15761/NDT.1000135.

44. Ming X, Stein TP, Barnes V, Rhodes N, Guo L (2012) Metabolic perturbance in autism spectrum disorders: a metabolomics study. J Proteome Res
11: 5856-5862.

45. Bala KA, DoÄŸan M, Mutluer T, Kaba S, Aslan O, et al. (2016) Plasma
amino acid profile in autism spectrum disorder (ASD). Eur Rev Med Pharmacol Sci 20: 923-929.

46. Geier, D.A.; Kern, J.K.; Davis, G.; King, P.G.; Adams, J.B.; Young, J.L.;
Geier, M.R. A prospective double-blind, randomized clinical trial of
levocarnitine to treat autism spectrum disorders. Med. Sci. Monit. 2011, 17,
PI15–PI23.

47. Fahmy, S.F.; El-hamamsy, M.H.; Zaki, O.K.; Badary, O.A. L-Carnitine
supplementation improves the behavioral symptoms in autistic children.
Res. Autism Spectr. Disord. 2013, 7, 159–166.

48. Rossignol, D. A., & Frye, R. E. (2012). Mitochondrial dysfunction in autism
spectrum disorders: A systematic review and meta-analysis. Molecular
Psychiatry, 17(3), 290-314.

49. Sanctuary, M.R.; Kain, J.N.; Chen, S.Y.; Kalanetra, K.; Lemay, D.G.; Rose,
D.R.; Yang, H.T.; Tancredi, D.J.; German, J.B.; Slupsky, C.M.; et al. Pilot
study of probiotic/colostrum supplementation on gut function in children
with autism and gastrointestinal symptoms. PLoS ONE 2019, 14, e0210064.

50. Gvozdjakova A, Kucharska J, Ostatnikova D, Babinska K, Nakladal D,
Crane FL. Ubiquinol improves symptoms in children with autism. Oxid
Med Cell Longev, 2014;2014:798957.

51. Blackmer AB, Feinstein JA. Management of sleep disorders in children
with neurodevelopmental disorders: a review. Pharmacotherapy.
2016;36(1):84–98.

52. Rossignol DA, Frye RE. Melatonin in autism spectrum disorders. Curr
Clin Pharmacol. 2014;9(4):326-34.

53. Rossignol DA, Frye RE. Melatonin in autism spectrum disorders: a systematic review and meta-analysis. Dev Med Child Neurol. 2011;53(9):783-92.

54. Malow B, Adkins KW, McGrew SG, et al. Melatonin for sleep in children
with autism: a controlled trial examining dose, tolerability, and outcomes. J
Autism Dev Disord. 2012;42(8):1729-37. author reply 1738.

55. Wright B, Sims D, Smart S, et al. Melatonin versus placebo in children
with autism spectrum conditions and severe sleep problems not amenable
to behaviour management strategies: a randomised controlled crossover
trial. J Autism Dev Disord 2010; 41:175-184.

56. Wirojanan J, Jacquemont S, Diaz R, et al. The efficacy of melatonin for
sleep problems in children with autism, fragile X syndrome, or autism and
fragile X syndrome. J Clin Sleep Med 2009; 5:145-150.

57. Cortesi F, Giannotti F, Sebastiani T, Panunzi S, Valente D. Controlled-release melatonin, singly and combined with cognitive behavioural therapy, for persistent insomnia in children with autism spectrum disorders: a randomized placebo-controlled trial. J Sleep Res. 2012;21(6):700–9.

58. Blaylock RL, Strunecka A Immune-glutametric Dysfunction as A central Mechanism of the Autism Spectrum Disorders. Curr Med Chem 2009; 16:157-70.

59. Acuna-Castroviejo D, Escames G, Venegas C, Diaz-Casado ME, Lima-Cabello E, Lopez LC, et al. Extrapineal melatonin: sources, regulation, and potential functions. Cell Mol Life Sci 2014; 71: 2997-3025.

60. Grigg-Damberger M, Ralls F. Treatment strategies for complex behavioral insomnia in children with neurodevelopmental disorders. Curr Opin Pulm Med, 2013;19:616-625.

Chapter Twelve

1. Buie T, Campbell DB, Fuchs GJ 3rd, et al. Evaluation, diagnosis, and treatment of gastrointestinal disorders in individuals with ASDs: a consensus report. Pediatrics. 2010;125(Suppl 1):S1-S18.

2. Maenner MJ, Arneson CL, Levy SE, Kirby RS, Nicholas JS, Durkin MS. Brief report: association between behavioral features and gastrointestinal problems among children with autism spectrum disorder. J Autism Dev Disord. 2012;42(7):1520-1525.

3. Buie T, Fuchs GJ 3rd, Furuta GT, Kooros K, Levy J, Lewis JD, et al. Recommendations for evaluation and treatment of common gastrointestinal problems in children with ASDs. Pediatrics. 2010 January;125 Suppl 1: S19--29.

4. American Academy of Pediatrics, Subcommittee on Chronic Abdominal Pain. Chronic abdominal pain in children. Pediatrics. 2005;115(3):812-815.

5. Rossignol DA, Frye RE. Mitochondrial dysfunction in autism spectrum disorders: a systematic review and meta-analysis. Mol Psychiatry 2012; 17: 290-314.

6. Frye RE, Rossignol DA. Mitochondrial dysfunction can connect the diverse medical symptoms associated with autism spectrum disorders. Pediatr Res 2011; 69: 41R-7R.

7. Frye RE. Biomarkers of abnormal energy metabolism in children with autism spectrum disorder. N Am J Med Sci 2012; 5: 141-7.

8. Catalano P, Walker J (2018) Understanding Nasal Breathing: The Key to Evaluating and Treating Sleep Disordered Breathing in Adults and Children. Curr Trends Otolaryngol Rhinol: CTOR-121. DOI: 10.29011/ CTOR-121. 000021

9. Bonuck, K., T. Rao, and L. Xu. "Pediatric Sleep Disorders and Special Educational Need at 8 Years: A Population-Based Cohort Study." PEDIATRICS 130, no. 4 (October 1, 2012): 634–42. https://doi.org/10.1542/peds.2012-0392.

10. Bolte E. Autism and Clostridium tetani. Med Hypotheses 1998; 51:133-144.

11. Adams, J.B., Audhya, T., McDonough-Means, S., Rubin, R.A., Quig, D., Geis, E., et al., 2013. Toxicological status of children with autism vs. neurotypical children and the association with autism severity. Biol. Trace Elem. Res. 151 (2), 171-180.

12. Gorbach S, Chang T, Goldin B. Successful treatment of relapsing Clostridium difficile colitis with Lactobacillus GG. Lancet 1987; 2: 1519.

13. Shaw W. Increased urinary excretion of a 3-(3-hydroxyphenyl)-3-hydroxypropionic acid (HPHPA), an abnormal phenylalanine metabolite of Clostridia spp. in the gastrointestinal tract, in urine samples from patients with autism and schizophrenia. Nutr Neurosci 2010;13:135-43.

14. Mezzelani A, Landini M, Facchiano F, Raggi ME, Villa L, Molteni M, et al. Environment, dysbiosis, immunity and sex-specific susceptibility: a translational hypothesis for regressive autism pathogenesis. Nutr Neurosci 2015;18(4):14561. doi:10.1179/1476830513Y.0000000108.

15. Kaluzna-Czaplinska J, Blaszczyk S. The level of arabinitol in autistic children after probiotic therapy. Nutrition (2012) 28:1246.doi: 10.1016/j.nut.2011.08.002.

16. Tomova, Aleksandra & Marcincakova Husarova, Veronika & Lakatosova, Silvia & Bakos, Jan & Vlková, Barbora & Babinska, Katarina & Ostatníková, Daniela. (2014). Gastrointestinal microbiota in children with autism in Slovakia. Physiology & Behavior. 138. 10.1016/j.physbeh.2014.10.033.

17. Sandler RH, Finegold SM, Bolte ER et al. Short-term benefit from oral vancomycin treatment of regressive-onset autism. J Child Neurol 2000; 15:429-435.

18. Shaw W, Kassen E, Chaves E. Assessment of antifungal drug therapy in autism by measurement of suspected microbial metabolites in urine with gas chromatography-mass spectrometry. Clin Pract Alter Med 2000;1:1526.

Printed in Great Britain
by Amazon

26356639R00195